Key References in Endocrinology

AN ANNOTATED GUIDE

PERRY J. BLACKSHEAR, M.D., D.Phil.
Assistant Professor of Medicine
Harvard Medical School
Assistant in Medicine
Massachusetts General Hospital
Associate Investigator
Howard Hughes Medical Institute
Boston, Massachusetts

Churchill Livingstone
New York, Edinburgh, London, and Melbourne
1982

Distributed in the United Kingdom by Churchill Livingstone, Robert Stevenson House, 1-3 Baxter's Place, Leith Walk, Edinburgh EHI 3AF and by associated companies, branches and representatives throughout the world.

First published 1982
Printed in USA
ISBN 0-443-08210-3
7 6 5 4 3 2 1

Library of Congress Cataloging in Publication Data

Blackshear, Perry J.
Key references in endocrinology.

(Key references in internal medicine)
1. Endocrine glands—Diseases—Bibliography.
2. Endocrine glands—Diseases—Abstracts.
3. Clinical endocrinology—Bibliography. I. Title.
II. Series. [DNLM: 1. Endocrinology—Abstracts.
ZWK 100 B631k]
Z6664.E57B57 1982 [RC649] 016.6164 82-14662
ISBN 0-443-08210-3

Key References in Endocrinology

AN ANNOTATED GUIDE

Key References in Internal Medicine

AN ANNOTATED GUIDE

Editors
Perry J. Blackshear, M.D., D.Phil.
Richard D. Klausner, M.D.

VOLUMES

Key References in Cardiology: An Annotated Guide
JOHN F. SCHNEIDER, M.D.

Key References in Pulmonary Medicine: An Annotated Guide
LEONARD SONNE, M.D.

Key References in Nephrology: An Annotated Guide
JOSEPH V. BONVENTRE, M.D., PH.D.

Key References in Gastroenterology: An Annotated Guide
MARK S. McPHEE, M.D., JAMES M. RICHTER, M.D., AND R. JAMES KLINGENSTEIN, M.D.

Key References in Endocrinology: An Annotated Guide
PERRY J. BLACKSHEAR, M.D., D.PHIL.

Key References in Infectious Diseases: An Annotated Guide
FREDERICK S. SOUTHWICK, M.D., AND ROBERT T. SCHOOLEY, M.D.

Key References in Hematology and Oncology: An Annotated Guide
ROGER JAY KURLANDER, M.D.

Key References in Rheumatology: An Annotated Guide
RICHARD D. KLAUSNER, M.D., AND MALCOLM S. THALER, M.D.

Preface

One of the questions most frequently asked of a subspecialty consultant, at least by the medical housestaff and medical students, is: "Have you got any good references on ———?" The idea for this series arose when, as house officers, we did not always get satisfactory answers to this question. We thought that a collection of key references in internal medicine, selected by recent graduates of subspecialty fellowship programs, might be of value, especially to busy house officers and medical students who rarely have the time for a careful literature search. Instead of a simple list of references, we decided to include brief annotations to give the reader some idea of each article's content; the number of references cited in each paper is noted at the end of each annotation, to give the reader some idea of whether or not it is worth looking up for further literature sources. Finally, we wished to include a few references on even the most obscure topics, rather than concentrate exclusively on common diseases, since the literature pertaining to rare subjects is often rather obscure itself.

As the project progressed, it became apparent that each author had his own idea about how to interpret Dr. Klausner's and my initial general guidelines. This is one of the reasons for the considerable heterogeneity among the sections in length and content of annotation, writing style, and selection and number of references. These concerns have all been left up to the individual author; our function as editors has been largely one of correcting spelling and grammar, suggesting the addition of topics of interest, and haranguing the contributors about deadlines. In general, they are responsible for the content of their volumes.

In *Key References in Endocrinology,* I have tried to collect what I believe to be the most interesting, useful, or, in other ways, "key" references in the subspecialty. The most recent references are from early 1982; however, my experience was that many of the most useful papers were written several years ago. No attempt has been made to establish chronological priorities, and, in general, the most recent complete reviews of a subject are listed. I apologize in advance for any omissions and welcome (polite!) suggestions about key references that could have been listed. Finally, although pertinent data from the papers often are described in the annotations, these data are not meant to supplant a trip to the library to look up the original.

I would like to thank Lewis Reines of Churchill Livingstone for his enthusiasm and encouragement as the project progressed; the other authors of this series, who worked long and hard and eventually did finish their volumes; Kathy O'Neill for typing the manuscript; and my wife for putting up with me during many long stints in the library.

Perry J. Blackshear, M.D., D.Phil.

Key References in Endocrinology

AN ANNOTATED GUIDE

Key References in Endocrinology

HYPOTHALAMIC-PITUITARY DISORDERS

Physiology and Diagnosis

Edwards CRW and Besser GM: Diseases of the hypothalamus and pituitary gland. ***Clin Endocrinol Metab,*** **3:475–505, 1974.**
A practical guide to the diagnosis of several common disorders of the pituitary gland, including acromegaly, hypopituitarism, dwarfism, galactorrhea and diabetes insipidus. 77 refs.

Locke W: Control of anterior pituitary function. ***Arch Intern Med,*** **138:1,541–1,545, 1978.**
A nice, short review of drugs, conditions and hormones affecting anterior pituitary secretion. 15 refs.

Reichlin S: Regulation of the hypophysiotropic secretions of the brain. ***Arch Intern Med,*** **135:1,350–1,361, 1975.**
A brief and readable review of this complex topic. 75 refs.

Vale W, Rivier C and Brown M: Regulatory peptides of the hypothalamus. ***Ann Rev Physiol,*** **39:473–527, 1977.**
A detailed review of hypothalamic releasing factors and related peptides. 537 refs.

VanWyk JJ and Underwood LE: Relation between growth hormone and somatomedin. ***Ann Rev Med,*** **26:427–441, 1975.**
A detailed review of what was known of the somatomedins in 1975. 96 refs.

Root AW, Reiter EO and Weisman Y: Current status and clinical application of the hypothalamic hormones. ***Adv Pediatr,*** **23:151–211, 1976.**
A detailed review of the physiology and clinical applications of the hypothalamic releasing hormones, not only in children. 349 refs.

Sinding C and Robinson AG: A review of neurophysins. ***Metabolism,*** **26:1,355–1,370, 1977.**
A brief review of what is known about these substances with comments on the absence of a known biologic function for them. 94 refs.

Robinson AG: The neurophysins in health and disease. ***Clin Endocrinol Metab,*** **6:261–275, 1977.**
A concise review of these mysterious posterior pituitary hormones. 42 refs.

Edwards CRW: Vasopressin and oxytocin in health and disease. ***Clin Endocrinol Metab,*** **6:223–259, 1977.**
An extensive review of physiology and pathology of these posterior pituitary hormones. About 240 refs.

Robertson GL: The regulation of vasopressin function in health and disease. ***Recent Prog Horm Res,*** **33:333–385, 1977.**
An extensive review of the regulation of vasopressin secretion and its physiological actions in man, with brief comments on diabetes insipidus and syndrome of inappropriate antidiuretic hormone secretion (SIADH). 98 refs.

Besser GM and Mortimer CH: Hypothalamic regulatory hormones: A review. ***J Clin Pathol,*** **27:173–184, 1974.**
A brief review of the 1974 status of the hypothalamic releasing factors, by two prominent workers in the field. 99 refs.

Guillemin R and Gerich JE: Somatostatin: Physiological and clinical significance. ***Ann Rev Med,*** **27:379–388, 1976.**
A very brief review of the possible clinical significance of somatostatin with special emphasis on its usefulness as a sup-

pressor of growth hormone, insulin and glucagon secretion. 81 refs.

Wurtman RJ and Moskowitz MA: The pineal organ. ***N Engl J Med,*** **296:1,329–1,333; 1,383–1,386, 1977.**
A review of what little is known of this tiny organ, with emphasis on the regulation and importance of melatonin secretion. 83 refs.

Frohman LA: Clinical neuropharmacology of hypothalamic releasing factors. ***N Engl J Med,*** **286:1,391–1,397, 1972.**
A brief, readable, but now somewhat dated review of this subject. 76 refs.

Frohman LA and Stachura ME: Neuropharmacologic control of neuroendocrine function in man. ***Metabolism,*** **24:211–234, 1975.**
An extensive review of the peptidergic regulation of pituitary hormone secretion, with emphasis on the possible role of neurotransmitters in both hypothalamic and pituitary hormone release. 160 refs.

Weitzman ED: Circadian rhythms and episodic hormone secretion in man. ***Ann Rev Med,*** **27:225–243, 1976.**
An interesting review of the biologic rhythms of pituitary hormone secretion, emphasizing the physiologic utility of these rhythms, and their abnormalities in pathologic states. 112 refs.

Cohen KL: Metabolic, endocrine and drug-induced interference with pituitary function tests: A review. ***Metabolism,*** **26:1,165–1,177, 1977.**
A brief but important review of factors which can interfere with pituitary function testing, including endocrine and psychiatric disorders and drugs. 90 refs.

Spark RF: Simplified assessment of pituitary-adrenal reserve. Measurement of serum 11-deoxycortisol and cortisol after metyrapone. ***Ann Intern Med,*** **75:717–723, 1971.**
This modification of the standard metyrapone test was successful in delineating subnormal ACTH responses in patients with hypopituitarism (15) or acromegaly (12) as well as patients on long-term steroid therapy (13). The response was normal in eight patients with enlarged sellas but no endocrinopathies. 18 refs.

Harsoulis P, Marshall JC, Kuku SF et al.: Combined test for assessment of anterior pituitary function. ***Br Med J,*** **4:326–329, 1973.**

A brief description of what has become an extremely useful and timesaving test in assessing anterior pituitary function: The combined TRH/insulin/LHRH test, here performed in 24 subjects. No differences were found when the tests were performed separately or together. 23 refs.

Eddy RL, Gilliland PF, Ibarra JD et al.: Human growth hormone release: Comparison of provocative test procedures. *Am J Med,* 56:179–185, 1974.
L-dopa and insulin tolerance tests were more effective in evoking a normal growth hormone response than arginine, glucagon or vasopressin in 20 normal volunteers. 39 refs.

Weisberg LA, Zimmerman EA and Frantz AG: Diagnosis and evaluation of patients with an enlarged sella turcica. *Am J Med,* 61:590–596, 1976.
Of 100 patients referred for evaluation of an enlarged sella, 75 had no visual symptoms. Of these, 27 had intrasellar tumors, 25 had empty sellas and 13 had an extrasellar process. 10 further patients had no pneumoencephalogram but had no symptoms up to 3 years later. 27 refs.

Doyle F and McLachlan M: Radiological aspects of pituitary-hypothalamic disease. *Clin Endocrinol Metab,* 6:53–81, 1977.
An informative review of useful radiologic procedures in the evaluation of pituitary lesions, including CT scans and angiography. A brief discussion of other space-occupying pituitary lesions is included. 83 refs.

DiChiro G and Nelson KB: The volume of the sella turcica. *Am J Roentgenol,* 87:989–1,008, 1962.
An early but still useful study of radiographic determination of sellar volume, compared with pituitary gland and sellar volume in 66 cadavers. 57 refs.

Naldich TP, Pinto RS, Kushner MJ et al.: Evaluation of sellar and parasellar masses by computed tomography. *Radiology,* 120:91–99, 1976.
CT scans from 65 patients with parasellar masses (including 26 pituitary adenomas) were evaluated. The authors feel that . . . "CT has proved completely reliable for detecting or ruling out the presence of a suprasellar mass. . . ." 15 refs.

Gross CE, Binet EF and Esguerra JV: Metrizamide cisternography in the evaluation of pituitary adenomas and the empty sella syndrome. *J Neurosurg,* 50:472–476, 1979.
A brief description of the use of metrizamide cisternography in the evaluation of pituitary mass lesions in three patients.

Because of its convenience and lack of side effects, this test is rapidly replacing the pneumoencephalogram. 9 refs.

Nabarro JDN: Pituitary surgery for endocrine disorders. *Clin Endocrinol,* 13:285–298, 1980.
The author reviews the indications for various types of pituitary surgery in the treatment of pituitary adenomas. He includes comments on preoperative radiologic evaluation, as well as on intraoperative steroid coverage and postoperative endocrine assessment. 79 refs.

Wilson CB and Dempsey LC: Transsphenoidal microsurgical removal of 250 pituitary adenomas. *J Neurosurg,* 48:13–22, 1978.
The authors present the results of 250 transsphenoidal procedures in patients with pituitary adenomas. There was one postoperative death. Major or minor CSF rhinorrhea was noted in 6.4 percent; bacterial meningitis in 2 percent; mental change in 1.6 percent; and persistent total or partial diabetes insipidus in 5.6 percent. 26 refs.

Teears RJ and Silverman EM: Clinicopathologic review of 88 cases of carcinoma metastatic to the pituitary gland. *Cancer,* 36:216–220, 1975.
In 88 patients with carcinoma metastatic to the pituitary, the anterior lobe alone was involved in only 13.6 percent. The posterior lobe was involved in 69 percent, although only 7 percent of patients had diabetes insipidus. Most common primaries were breast (66 percent), lung (13 percent) and stomach (7.5 percent) in women; lung (63 percent), prostate (9 percent) and bladder (6 percent) in men. 11 refs.

Galactorrhea-Amenorrhea Syndromes

Frantz AG: Prolactin. *N Engl J Med,* 298:201–207, 1978.
A concise review of prolactin physiology and pathophysiology. 17 refs.

Kleinberg DL, Noel GL and Frantz AG: Galactorrhea: A study of 235 cases, including 48 with pituitary tumors. *N Engl J Med,* 296:589–600, 1977.
An excellent discussion of the causes of galactorrhea in 235 patients. 20 percent had pituitary tumors; 34 percent of patients with associated amenorrhea had tumors. 32 percent had "idiopathic" galactorrhea with menses. 58 refs.

Franks S, Murray MAF, Jequier AM et al.: Incidence and significance of hyperprolactinemia in women with amenorrhea. *Clin Endocrinol,* 4:597–607, 1975.

Prolactin levels were normal in 106 amenorrheic patients with primary ovarian failure, anorexia nervosa, marked obesity and post-pill amenorrhea. Elevated prolactins were found in 13 patients (12 percent) with pituitary tumors; 8 of 40 patients with "functional" amenorrhea had elevated prolactins. 40 refs.

Gomez F, Reyes FI and Faiman C: Non-puerperal galactorrhea and hyperprolactinemia: Clinical findings, endocrine features and therapeutic responses in 56 cases. ***Am J Med,*** **62:648–660, 1977.**
Of 56 patients studied, 5 had elevated prolactin levels and normal skull x-rays; they later developed abnormal sellar films within 5 years, indicating enlargement of a pituitary adenoma. 78 refs.

Davajan V, Kletzky O, March CM et al.: The significance of galactorrhea in patients with normal menses, oligomenorrhea and secondary amenorrhea. ***Am J Obstet Gynecol,*** **130:894–900, 1978.**
149 women with galactorrhea were studied, 32 of whom had normal menses. Three had hypothyroidism. 62 percent had elevated prolactins. 9 women with abnormal sellar tomograms had normal prolactins; of 32 patients with normal menses, 19 had elevated prolactins. 18 refs.

Jacobs HS, Franks S, Murray MAF et al.: Clinical and endocrine features of hyperprolactinaemic amenorrhoea. ***Clin Endocrinol,*** **5:439–454, 1976.**
Studies were performed on 35 women with amenorrhea and hyperprolactinemia. 12 had x-ray evidence of pituitary tumors. Galactorrhea was present in 30 percent. Withdrawal bleeding after a progestin occurred in only 2 of 21 patients, indicating a low estrogen status. Responses to TRH were flat in all patients. 33 refs.

Boyd AE III, Reichlin S and Turksoy RN: Galactorrhea-amenorrhea syndrome: Diagnosis and therapy. ***Ann Intern Med,*** **87:165–175, 1977.**
Patients with amenorrhea and galactorrhea (7 with known pituitary adenomas and 18 with normal x-rays) were compared with 8 normal women. Several patients with the "idiopathic" syndrome had elevated prolactins. Most (but not all) patients with adenomas had flat TRH responses. 50 refs.

Swanson JA, Jacoby CG, Sherman BM et al.: Evaluation of the pituitary. Patients with suspected prolactin-producing tumors. ***Obstet Gynecol,*** **52:67–72, 1978.**

27 of 100 patients referred for the evaluation of galactorrhea/amenorrhea had suspicious skull films; 22 of these had hyperprolactinemia. This paper provides a nice discussion of pituitary radiology and anatomy. 13 refs.

Cowden EA, Ratcliffe JG, Thomson JA et al.: Tests of prolactin secretion in diagnosis of prolactinomas. *Lancet,* 1:1,155–1,158, 1979.
14 patients with histologically proven prolactinomas were studied. All had amenorrhea; 29 percent had galactorrhea. Half the patients had normal sellar tomograms; but all displayed a flat response to TRH and metoclopramide stimulation. 24 refs.

Healy DL, Pepperell RJ, Stockdale J et al.: Pituitary autonomy in hyperprolactinemic secondary amenorrhea: Results of hypothalamic pituitary testing. *J Clin Endocrinol Metab,* 44:809–819, 1977.
27 patients with secondary amenorrhea were studied. Nine had normal responses to TRH and metoclopramide, and normal baseline prolactin levels. 18 had high baseline prolactin levels, and were unresponsive to TRH and metoclopramide; 15 of these had galactorrhea. Bromocryptine, L-dopa and LHRH tests were equivocal. 36 refs.

Friesen HG and Tolis G: The use of bromocryptine in the galactorrhea-amenorrhea syndromes: The Canadian cooperative study. *Clin Endocrinol,* suppl., 6:91S–99S, 1977.
Bromocryptine was used to treat 79 women with galactorrhea-amenorrhea, diagnosed as "functional" (44 patients), or secondary to microadenomas (18 patients), macroadenomas (7 patients) or stalk surgery (9 patients). Bromocryptine caused sustained decreases in prolactin in all patients; principal side effects were nausea, vomiting, headache and dizziness. 13 refs.

Thorner MO, McNeilly AS, Hagan C et al.: Long-term treatment of galactorrhea and hypogonadism with bromocryptine. *Br Med J,* 2:419–422, 1974.
The authors treated 17 women and 4 men with galactorrhea and hypogonadism with bromocryptine. Prolactin levels decreased; 18 patients developed normal gonadal status. Side effects of bromocryptine were dyspepsia and nausea in five patients. 27 refs.

Thorner MO, Martin WH, Rogol AD et al.: Rapid regression of pituitary prolactinomas during bromocriptine treatment. *J Clin Endocrinol Metab,* 51:438–445, 1980.

Large prolactinomas in two patients regressed rapidly and markedly on bromocryptine therapy, with improvement of clinical symptoms. The authors raise the intriguing question of whether medical therapy alone is indicated for large prolactinomas. 41 refs.

Hardy J: Transsphenoidal microsurgery of the normal and pathological pituitary. ***Clin Neurosurg,*** **16:185–217, 1969.**
A classic article describing the now standard surgical approach to pituitary microadenomas. 50 refs.

Carter JN, Tyson JE, Tolis G et al.: Prolactin-secreting tumors and hypogonadism in 22 men. ***N Engl J Med,*** **299:847–852, 1978.**
22 men with hyperprolactinemic hypogonadism were studied, 13 receiving bromocryptine and 17 operation or radiation or both. Bromocryptine improved symptoms in many patients unresponsive to other forms of pituitary tumor ablation. 27 refs.

Tucker H St G, Grubb SR, Wigand JP et al: Galactorrhea-amenorrhea syndromes: Follow-ups of 45 patients after pituitary tumor removal. ***Ann Intern Med,*** **94:302–307, 1981.**
Prolactinomas were removed from 45 patients with galactorrea-amenorrhea. Follow-up an average of 3.1 years later showed that apparent cures were most common in patients with small, nonevasive tumors. Prolactin levels obtained 6 months post-operatively, but not earlier, apparently predicted cures. 13 refs.

Acromegaly

Merimee TJ and Rabin D: A survey of growth hormone secretion and action. ***Metabolism,*** **22:1,235–1,251, 1973.**
A complete review of the physiology of growth hormone secretion and action, now somewhat dated. 63 refs.

Cryer PE, Daughaday WH, Coxe WS and Avioli LV: Diagnosis and therapy of acromegaly. ***Arch Intern Med,*** **135:338–343, 1975.**
A brief review of the physiology of growth hormone secretion, and the diagnosis and therapy of acromegaly. 23 refs.

Haigler ED, Hershman JM and Meador CK: Pituitary gigantism. ***Arch Intern Med,*** **132:588–594, 1973.**
A case report and review of the literature on pituitary gigantism, differentiating this syndrome of growth hormone excess from acromegaly. 44 refs.

Roth J, Glick SM and Cuatrecasas P: Acromegaly and other disorders of growth hormone secretion. ***Ann Intern Med,*** **66:760–788, 1967.**
A review of early growth hormone measurements in acromegaly and other disorders of growth hormone secretion. 67 refs.

Earll JM, Sparks LL and Forsham PM: Glucose suppression of serum growth hormone in the diagnosis of acromegaly. ***JAMA,*** **201:628–630, 1967.**
The standard test in the diagnosis of acromegaly is described, the 100 gram oral glucose tolerance test. Growth hormone was completely suppressed in normal volunteers, but not in 15 patients with acromegaly 1 hour after glucose ingestion. 26 refs.

McLachlan MSF, Wright AD and Doyle FH: Plain film and tomographic assessment of the pituitary fossa in 140 acromegalic patients. ***Br J Radiol,*** **43:360–369, 1970.**
Sellar radiographs of 140 patients with acromegaly were evaluated. 55 percent showed gross abnormalities on plain films and 27 percent showed a double contour only; of the remaining 18 percent, smaller abnormalities were demonstrated only on tomography. 12 refs.

Quabbe H-J: Treatment of acromegaly by trans-sphenoidal operation, 90-yttrium implantation and bromocriptine: Results in 230 patients. ***Clin Endocrinol,*** **16:107–119, 1982.**
In a prospective study of 230 patients with acromegaly treated by various means, the authors concluded that the best results were achieved with trans-sphenoidal surgery, where the best results were obtained with smaller tumors. The other modalities were less effective, had more complications, or both. 32 refs.

Wass JAH, Thorner MO, Morris DV et al.: Long-term treatment of acromegaly with bromocryptine. ***Br Med J,*** **1:875–878, 1977.**
Bromocryptine (10–60 mg/day) was given to 73 patients with acromegaly for 3 to 25 months. Most patients showed symptomatic improvement; however, growth hormone levels fell to less than 5 ng/ml in only 15 patients. Common side effects included constipation, digital vasospasm, nausea and dry mouth. 15 refs.

Sachdev Y, Gomez-Pan A, Tunbridge WMG et al.: Bromocryptine therapy in acromegaly. ***Lancet,*** **2:1,164–1,168, 1975.**
21 acromegalic patients were treated with bromocryptine,

which substantially decreased serum growth hormone levels in 12 patients when used in doses of 20 to 40 mg/day. Several patients did not respond. 30 refs.

Atkinson RL, Becker DP, Martins AN et al.: Acromegaly: Treatment by transsphenoidal microsurgery. *JAMA,* 233:1,279–1,283, 1975.
7 of 9 patients undergoing transsphenoidal surgery for previously untreated acromegaly experienced decreased growth hormone levels; 6 of 7 patients previously treated with other forms of therapy experienced decreases of growth hormone to less than 10 ng/ml. Other pituitary hormones were quite commonly affected in this early series. 35 refs.

Arafah BM, Brodkey JS, Kaufman B et al.: Transsphenoidal microsurgery in the treatment of acromegaly and gigantism. *J Clin Endocrinol Metab,* 50:578–585, 1980.
28 patients underwent attempted resection of a growth hormone secreting tumor. 11 patients were thought to be cured, with 2 more cured but hypopituitary. 14 of 15 patients not cured had extrasellar extension at surgery, in contrast to 2 of 13 patients considered cured. 32 refs.

Kjellberg RN, Shintani A, Frantz AG and Kliman B: Proton-beam therapy in acromegaly. *N Engl J Med,* 278:689–695, 1968.
Of 22 patients with acromegaly, 14 were followed for 2 to 36 months. Growth hormone levels fell markedly in eight; panhypopituitarism and serious visual loss occurred in one patient each. 41 refs.

Roth J, Gorden P and Brace K: Efficacy of conventional pituitary radiation in acromegaly. *N Engl J Med,* 282:1,385–1,391, 1970.
20 patients with acromegaly were treated with conventional supravoltage radiation (4,000 R). The mean decrease in growth hormone levels was 51 percent after 1 year; however, relatively few values were below 5 ng/ml. 38 refs.

Goldfine ID: Medical treatment of acromegaly. *Annu Rev Med,* 29:407–415, 1978.
A short review of recent advances in the pharmacology of growth hormone secretion. 49 refs.

McGuffin WL, Sherman BM, Roth J et al.: Acromegaly and cardiovascular disorders. A prospective study. *Ann Intern Med,* 81:11–18, 1974.
Of 57 patients with acromegaly, hypertension was present in 13; 9 other patients had heart disease, including 4 with ar-

rythmias and 9 with congestive heart failure of varying etiologies. Cardiomegaly was detectable clinically only in patients with congestive failure or hypertension, but was present in all autopsied patients. The authors failed to find a characteristic form of heart disease in acromegaly. 33 refs.

O'Duffy JD, Randall RV and MacCarty CS: Median neuropathy (carpal tunnel syndrome) in acromegaly. ***Ann Intern Med,*** **78:379–383, 1973.**
Of 100 patients with acromegaly, 35 had carpal tunnel syndrome. It was usually associated with active disease, and cleared with successful treatment. 16 refs.

Harrison BDW, Millhouse KA, Harrington M and Nabarro JDN: Lung function in acromegaly. ***Q J Med,*** **47:517–532, 1978.**
Lung function was evaluated in 30 patients with acromegaly; 8 were excluded because of kyphosis or pulmonary hypertension. The incidences of increased total lung capacity, small airway narrowing and extrathoracic airway narrowing were high, and related to duration of disease. 26 refs.

Pickett JBE III, Layzer RB, Levin SR et al.: Neuromuscular complications of acromegaly. ***Neurology,*** **25:638–645, 1975.**
Neuromuscular evaluation was performed in 17 acromegalic patients. Nine patients had a characteristic myopathy consisting of proximal weakness with normal biopsy and enzymes; eight patients had carpal tunnel syndrome. Both improved after therapy. 47 refs.

Nelson's Syndrome (See Also Cushing's Disease)

Cohen KL, Noth RH and Pechinski T: Incidence of pituitary tumors following adrenalectomy. ***Arch Intern Med,*** **138:575–579, 1978.**
10 probable pituitary adenomas were detected in 21 patients who had undergone bilateral adrenalectomy for Cushing's syndrome. The mean time from adrenalectomy to diagnosis was 6½ years. 14 refs.

Hopwood NJ and Kenny FM: Incidence of Nelson's syndrome after adrenalectomy for Cushing's disease in children. ***Am J Dis Child,*** **131:1,353–1,356, 1977.**
31 children were evaluated 1 to 5½ years after adrenalectomy for Cushing's syndrome. Hyperpigmentation was noted in 58 percent; sella enlargement in 25 percent and documented pituitary adenomas in 18 percent. 24 refs.

Moore TJ, Dluhy RG, Williams GH et al.: Nelson's syndrome: Frequency, prognosis and effect of prior pituitary irradiation. *Ann Intern Med,* 85:731–734, 1976.
The authors followed 120 patients 2 to 20 years after adrenalectomy for Cushing's syndrome. ACTH-secreting pituitary tumors developed in 8 percent, being diagnosed 6 months to 16 years post-adrenalectomy. In this series, pituitary irradiation did not prevent the development of pituitary tumors. 21 refs.

Nelson DH, Meakin JW and Thorn GW: ACTH-producing tumors following adrenalectomy for Cushing's syndrome. *Ann Intern Med,* 52:560–569, 1960.
An early description of 10 patients with this syndrome. All were deeply pigmented, and most had markedly elevated ACTH levels. Most of these patients had responded to exogenous ACTH prior to adrenalectomy. 8 refs.

Syndrome of Inappropriate Antidiuretic Hormone Secretion (SIADH)

Cooke CR, Turin MD and Walker WG: The syndrome of inappropriate antidiuretic hormone secretion (SIADH): Pathophysiologic mechanisms in solute and volume regulation. *Medicine,* 58:240–251, 1979.
Sodium and water balance studies were performed in eight patients with SIADH of varying causes. 59 refs.

Bartter FC and Schwartz WB: The syndrome of inappropriate secretion of antidiuretic hormone. *Am J Med,* 42:790–806, 1967.
A classic review by the authors of the first description of the syndrome, with emphasis on the differential diagnosis of hyponatremic states. 154 refs.

Carter NW, Rector FC Jr. and Seldin DW: Hyponatremia in cerebral disease resulting from the inappropriate secretion of antidiuretic hormone. *N Engl J Med,* 264:67–72, 1961.
Two patients with hyponatremia from cerebral disease were studied; the cause was inappropriate secretion of ADH in both. 17 refs.

Rosenow EC III, Segar WE and Zehr JE: Inappropriate antidiuretic hormone secretion in pneumonia. *Mayo Clin Proc,* 47:169–174, 1972.
Three patients with SIADH resulting from bacterial or viral pneumonia are described; the authors review the published cases of SIADH and pulmonary infection. 40 refs.

Miller M and Moses AM: Drug-induced states of impaired water excretion. ***Kidney Int,*** **10:96–103, 1976.**
A brief but thorough review of drugs known to cause hyponatremia. 102 refs.

Fichman MR, Vorherr H, Kleeman CR and Telfer N: Diuretic-induced hyponatremia. ***Ann Intern Med,*** **75:853–863, 1971.**
25 patients with diuretic-induced hyponatremia were studied; 10 of 10 patients with this syndrome showed elevated bioassayable vasopressin activity. Hypokalemia apparently potentiates vasopressin release in this syndrome, which is corrected by stopping the diuretic. 32 refs.

Vorherr H, Massry SG, Fallet R et al.: Antidiuretic principle in tuberculous lung tissue of a patient with pulmonary tuberculosis and hyponatremia. ***Ann Intern Med,*** **72:383–387, 1970.**
A compound with potent antidiuretic activity was isolated from tuberculous but not normal sections of lung from a patient with advanced tuberculosis and SIADH. 17 refs.

Padfield PL, Morton JJ, Brown JJ et al.: Plasma arginine vasopressin in the syndrome of antidiuretic hormone excess associated with bronchogenic carcinoma. ***Am J Med,*** **61:825–831, 1976.**
Of 17 patients with SIADH and bronchogenic carcinoma, plasma arginine vasopressin levels were above normal limits in 13. Vasopressin levels were also slightly higher than controls in 14 patients with bronchogenic carcinoma but without SIADH. 37 refs.

Nolph KD and Schrier RW: Sodium, potassium and water metabolism in the syndrome of inappropriate antidiuretic hormone secretion. ***Am J Med,*** **49:534–545, 1970.**
These authors describe detailed physiologic studies of sodium, potassium and water balance in a patient with SIADH secondary to an organic brain syndrome, with emphasis on renal mechanisms. 19 refs.

Forrest JN, Cox M, Hong C et al.: Superiority of demeclocycline over lithium in the treatment of chronic syndrome of inappropriate secretion of antidiuretic hormone. ***N Engl J Med,*** **298:173–177, 1978.**
10 patients with hyponatremia and inappropriate urine hyperosmolality despite fluid restriction were treated with demeclocycline (600–1,200 mg/day). This resulted in normal serum sodiums despite normal water intake in all patients within 2 weeks. Lithium was far less effective and poorly tolerated. 22 refs.

Hantman D, Rossier B, Zohlman R and Schrier R: Rapid correction of hyponatremia in the syndrome of inappropriate secretion of antidiuretic hormone. An alternative treatment to hypertonic saline. ***Ann Intern Med,*** **78:870–875, 1973.**
Five patients with SIADH received simultaneous rapid furosemide diuresis and electrolyte replacement. This was effective in rapidly restoring serum sodium to normal levels; it appears to be a reasonable alternative to hypertonic saline in hypervolemic patients. 28 refs.

Diabetes Insipidus

Hays RM: Antidiuretic hormone. ***N Engl J Med,*** **295:659–665, 1976.**
A short review of the synthesis, secretion, pharmacology and cellular actions of vasopressin. 26 refs.

Moses AM, Miller M and Streeten DHP: Pathophysiologic and pharmacologic alterations in the release and action of ADH. ***Metabolism,*** **25:697–721, 1976.**
The causes, diagnostic tests and treatments of diabetes insipidus and syndrome of inappropriate ADH release are reviewed in this paper, with new data from two large series of patients. The physiology of ADH is also reviewed. 164 refs.

Andreoli TE and Schafer JA: Some considerations of the role of antidiuretic hormone in water homeostasis. ***Recent Prog Horm Res,*** **33:387–434, 1977.**
A detailed review of biophysical aspects of renal water regulation by vasopressin. About 146 refs.

Price JD and Lanener RW: Serum and urine osmolalities in the differential diagnosis of polyuric states. ***J Clin Endocrinol Metab,*** **26:143–148, 1966.**
The authors describe the 8-hour water deprivation test, a useful diagnostic maneuver in the differentiation of diabetes insipidus from psychogenic polydipsia, in 29 normal men, 10 patients with diabetes insipidus and 2 with psychogenic polydipsia. 6 refs.

Berl T, Anderson RJ, McDonald KM and Schrier RW: Clinical disorders of water metabolism. ***Kidney Int,*** **10:117–132, 1976.**
A complete review of practical, clinical considerations in the diagnosis and management of diabetes insipidus and hyponatremic states. 138 refs.

Leaf A: Neurogenic diabetes insipidus. ***Kidney Int,*** **15:572–580, 1976.**

A short but recent review of this subject, with a discussion of anatomical considerations. 20 refs.

Miller M, Dalakos T, Moses AM et al.: Recognition of partial defects in antidiuretic hormone secretion. ***Ann Intern Med,*** **73:721–729, 1970.**
The authors describe 13 patients with partial diabetes insipidus, as determined by their response to water deprivation and further urine concentration after vasopressin injection. They discuss the usefulness of these tests in the diagnosis of polyuric states. 14 refs.

Singer I and Forrest JN Jr.: Drug-induced states of nephrogenic diabetes insipidus. ***Kidney Int,*** **10:82–95, 1976.**
Drug-induced nephrogenic diabetes insipidus is reviewed with emphasis on lithium, tetracyclines, sulfonylureas and methoxyfluorane. 88 refs.

Shacart WA and Jackson I: Management of diabetes insipidus in neurosurgical patients. ***J Neurosurg,*** **44:65–71, 1976.**
A short, practical review of the syndrome as it pertains to postoperative neurosurgical patients. 35 refs.

Robinson AG: DDAVP in the treatment of central diabetes insipidus. ***N Engl J Med,*** **294:507–511, 1976.**
Eight patients with complete central diabetes insipidus were treated with DDAVP, a synthetic analogue of vasopressin. Intranasal administration produced 8 to 20 hours of antidiuresis; side effects were nonexistent. This agent may replace available forms of vasopressin as standard therapy in central diabetes insipidus. 35 refs.

Webster B and Bain J: Antidiuretic effect and complications of chlorpropamide therapy in diabetes insipidus. ***J Clin Endocrinol Metab,*** **30:215–227, 1970.**
Chlorpropamide was used to treat 11 patients with central or idiopathic diabetes insipidus; in 5, hydrochlorothiazide was needed for full control. No effect was noted in one patient with nephrogenic diabetes insipidus. Hypoglycemia was a troublesome side effect. 20 refs.

Hypopituitarism

Sheehan HL and Summers VK: The syndrome of hypopituitarism. ***Q J Med,*** **18:319–356, 1949.**
A classic clinical description of the features of panhypopituitarism, as well as an exhaustive catalogue of its possible causes. Postpartem pituitary necrosis is also discussed. 307 refs.

Hall R: Diagnosis and management of hypopituitarism. ***J R Coll Physicians,*** **7:19–33, 1972.**
A complete review of partial and complete panhypopituitarism in a sometimes inaccessible journal. The etiologies and clinical features of the various syndromes are considered in detail. 38 refs.

Odell WD: Isolated deficiencies of anterior pituitary hormones: Symptoms and diagnosis. ***JAMA,*** **197:1,006–1,016, 1966.**
An interesting review of several rare syndromes, including isolated ACTH, TSH, growth hormone and gonadotropin deficiencies. Prolactin deficiency has since been described. 52 refs.

Goodman HG, Brambach MM and Kaplan SL: Growth and growth hormone. II: A comparison of isolated growth hormone deficiency and multiple pituitary hormone deficiencies in 35 patients with idiopathic hypopituitary dwarfism. ***N Engl J Med,*** **278:57–68, 1968.**
35 patients with idiopathic hypopituitary dwarfism were found to have heterogeneous hormone deficiencies: 16 had isolated growth hormone deficiency, while the others had multiple pituitary hormone deficiencies. Hypoglycemia was common in these patients; the dwarfism appeared nonfamilial. 79 refs.

Lombardi G, Minozzi M, Faggiano M et al.: Plasma immunoreactive T_3, TSH and ACTH before and after provocative tests in idiopathic hypopituitary dwarfism. ***J Clin Endocrinol Metab,*** **40:143–151, 1975.**
Eight patients with this disease were studied with provocative testing; all had disorders of TSH and ACTH secretion as well as growth hormone. 21 refs.

Samaan NA, Bakdash MM, Caderao JB et al.: Hypopituitarism after external irradiation. Evidence for both hypothalamic and pituitary origin. ***Ann Intern Med,*** **83:771–777, 1975.**
15 patients who had had radiotherapy for nasopharyngeal carcinoma were evaluated. 12 had evidence of hypothalamic dysfunction, 7 had hypopituitarism and 3 had primary hypothyroidism. 31 refs.

Stuart CA, Neelon FA and Lebovitz HE: Hypothalamic insufficiency: The cause of hypopituitarism in sarcoidosis. ***Ann Intern Med,*** **88:589–594, 1978.**
10 patients are described with severe sarcoidosis and hypopituitarism; however, 9 of these patients responded to TRH and LHRH, indicating that the disorder was primarily one of

hypothalamic dysfunction. Prolactin was elevated in six patients. 42 refs.

Parks JS, Tenore A, Bongiovanni AM and Kirkland RT: Familial hypopituitarism with large sella turcica. ***N Engl J Med,*** **298:698–702, 1978.**
Three siblings are described with short stature, full sellae and panhypopituitarism, a new syndrome which should be considered in the investigation of pituitary insufficiency in children. 20 refs.

Speckart PF, Nicoloff JT and Bethune JE: Screening for adrenocortical insufficiency with cosyntropin (synthetic ACTH). ***Arch Intern Med,*** **128:701–736, 1971.**
24 patients with various disorders were screened for adrenocortical insufficiency using this test; it was useful in separating primary or secondary hypoadrenalism from other disease states, and was much more convenient than an ACTH infusion. 12 refs.

Butler PWP and Besser GM: Pituitary adrenal function in severe depressive illness. ***Lancet,*** **1:1,234–1,236, 1968.**
Three patients with severe depression displayed elevated plasma and urinary corticosteroid concentrations, abnormal diurnal cortisol rhythms and some resistance to dexamethasone suppression; these abnormalities disappeared after treatment of the depression. 12 refs.

Merrimee TJ: Isolated growth hormone deficiency and related disorders. ***Annu Rev Med,*** **25:137–142, 1974.**
A brief discussion of what turns out to be a heterogeneous group of disorders. The author classifies growth hormone deficiency states into four types, based on the level of growth hormone in the blood, the presence of hypoglycemia and the "sulfation factor" response. 20 refs.

Odell WD and Swerdloff RS: Abnormalities of gonadal function in men. ***Clin Endocrinol,*** **8:149–180, 1978.**
The best recent review of this subject currently available, this paper describes the physiology of reproduction in men and its various disorders in an anatomical fashion: Hypothalamic, pituitary and primary gonadal disturbances. 160 refs.

Nowakowski H and Lenz W: Genetic aspects in male hypogonadism. ***Horm Metab Res,*** **17:53–95, 1961.**
A comprehensive review of genetically determined male hypogonadal disorders that is still current. 218 refs.

Mortimer CH, McNeilly AS, Fisher RA et al.: Gonadotropin-

releasing hormone therapy in hypogonadal males with hypothalamic or pituitary dysfunction. ***Br Med J,*** **4:617–621, 1974.**
Long-term 8-hourly subcutaneous injections of LHRH resulted in near-normal gonadotropin and androgen levels in 12 male patients with central hypoganadism. Sperm counts and potency also improved in several patients. 14 refs.

Bardin CW, Ross GT, Rifkind AB et al.: Studies of the pituitary-Leydig cell axis in young men with hypogonadotropic hypogonadism and hyposmia: Comparison with normal men, prepubertal boys and hypopituitary patients. ***J Clin Invest,*** **48:2,046–2,056, 1969.**
An early study of Kallmann's syndrome before the days of LHRH, showing low pituitary gonadotropin production and otherwise normal pituitary hormones in seven men. 42 refs.

Sparkes RS, Simpson RW and Paulsen CA: Familial hypogonadotropic hypogonadism with anosmia. ***Arch Intern Med,*** **121:534–538, 1968.**
Two brothers and one half-sister displayed the hallmarks of Kallmann's syndrome, while the mother was only slightly affected. The gonadotropin deficiency and anosmia were thought to be due to a hypothalamic disturbance. 23 refs.

McCann SM: Luteinizing-hormone-releasing hormone. ***N Engl J Med,*** **296:797–802, 1977.**
A nice brief review of the control of GNRH secretion and action. 11 refs.

Yoshimoto Y, Moridera K and Imura H: Restoration of normal pituitary gonadotropin reserve by administration of luteinizing-hormone-releasing-hormone in patients with hypogonadotropic hypogonadism. ***N Engl J Med,*** **292:242–245, 1975.**
The responses to LHRH stimulation were assessed before and after repeated intravenous LHRH infusions in 9 normal volunteers and 24 patients with hypogonadism of varying etiologies. This test proved useful in distinguishing between hypothalamic and hypopituitary hypogonadism. 21 refs.

The Empty Sella Syndrome

Jordan RM, Kendall JW and Kerber CW: The primary empty sella syndrome. Analysis of the clinical characteristics, radiographic features, pituitary function and cerebrospinal fluid adenohypophysial hormone concentrations. ***Am J Med,*** **62:569–580, 1977.**

These authors evaluated 12 patients with this syndrome and 247 cases from the literature. They found that the typical patient was an obese, multiparous woman with normal visual fields and endocrine status. An excellent literature review is included. 82 refs.

Neelon FA, Goree JA and Lebovitz AE: The primary empty sella: Clinical and radiographic and endocrine function. *Medicine,* 52:73–92, 1973.
30 patients were studied with this syndrome, 87 percent of whom were women, with a mean age of 48.6 years. Headache was present in 71 percent of patients. One patient had acromegaly, one had panhypopituitarism and three had partial pituitary hormone deficiency. 51 refs.

Domingue JN, Wing SD and Wilson CB: Coexisting pituitary adenomas and partially empty sellas. *J Neurosurg,* 48:23–28, 1978.
17 patients are described in whom both pituitary adenomas and empty sellas were present. Nine had acromegaly, and eight hyperprolactinemia. 23 refs.

Malarkey WB, Goodenow TJ and Lanese RR: Diurnal variation of prolactin secretion differentiates pituitary tumors from the primary empty sella syndrome. *Am J Med,* 69:886–890, 1980.
An interesting article in which 7 patients with empty sella syndrome were found to have normal diurnal prolactin patterns, in contrast to 16 patients with varyious pituitary tumors. This test may represent a noninvasive means of distinguishing between the empty sella syndrome and pituitary adenomas. 21 refs.

Anorexia Nervosa

Halmi KA: Anorexia nervosa: Recent investigations. *Annu Rev Med,* 29:137–148, 1978.
A brief review of the diagnosis of this disorder and recent metabolic and endocrine studies. 93 refs.

Kanis JA, Brown P, Fitzpatrick K et al.: Anorexia nervosa: A clinical, psychiatric and laboratory study. *Q J Med,* 43:321–338, 1974.
Detailed metabolic studies were carried out in 24 patients (all women) with anorexia nervosa, before and after psychiatric therapy. Most of the numerous endocrine abnormalities disappeared with successful therapy. 63 refs.

Vigersky RA, Loriaux DL, Andersen AE et al.: Anorexia ner-

vosa: Behavioral and hypothalamic aspects. ***Clin Endocrinol Metab*****, 5:517–535, 1976.**
32 patients with this disorder are described, 23 of which were evaluated endocrinologically. Mean basal growth hormone was high; basal gonadotropins and T_3 were low, but LH and FSH responded normally to LHRH, and the mean TSH response to TRH was also normal. Hypothalamic dysfunction, as manifested by disordered regulation of water and thermogenesis, was noted. 39 refs.

Hurd HP II, Palumbo PJ and Gharib H: Hypothalamic-endocrine dysfunction in anorexia nervosa. ***Mayo Clin Proc*****, 52:711–716, 1977.**
101 patients with anorexia nervosa were studied, 95 percent of whom were women. Amenorrhea was present in all women studied after menarche. Mean FSH, GH and cortisol levels were high; mean LH, estrogen and thyroxine levels were low, the last associated with a normal TSH. 79 refs.

Mecklenburg RS, Loriaux DL, Thompson RH et al.: Hypothalamic dysfunction in patients with anorexia nervosa. ***Medicine*****, 53:147–159, 1974.**
The hypothalamic-pituitary axes of five women with anorexia nervosa were evaluated. The authors concluded that the pituitary function was grossly normal, but that most patients showed evidence of hypothalamic dysfunction, including diabetes insipidus, impaired thermoregulation and insulin sensitivity. 98 refs.

McArthur JW, O'Loughlin KM, Beitins IZ et al.: Endocrine studies during the refeeding of young women with nutritional amenorrhea and infertility. ***Mayo Clin Proc*****, 51:607–616, 1976.**
Nine women with amenorrhea associated with weight loss were studied, none of whom had anorexia nervosa. LH levels were initially low; both LH levels and menses became normal when the patients' weight reached near-normal. 23 refs.

Pituitary Apopolexy

Rovit RL and Fein JM: Pituitary apoplexy: A review and reappraisal. ***J Neurosurg*****, 37:280–288, 1972.**
Nine cases of pituitary apoplexy are described, of which eight patients had chromophobe adenomas. Common symptoms included sudden headache, decreased consciousness, ophthalmoplegia, meningismus and visual field defects. CSF was bloody or xanthochromic in four of six cases. 57 refs.

Conomy JP, Ferguson JH, Brodkey JS and Mitsumoto H: Spon-

taneous infarction in pituitary tumors: Neurologic and therapeutic aspects. ***Neurology,*** **25:580–587, 1975.**
The authors describe two cases of this syndrome, and discuss the common symptoms, signs and available treatments for the disorder. 29 refs.

Pelkonen R, Kunsisto A, Salmi J et al.: Pituitary function after pituitary apoplexy. ***Am J Med,*** **65:773–778, 1978.**
Nine patients with various pituitary tumors were studied after spontaneous recovery from pituitary apoplexy; all developed some degree of pituitary hypofunction. Surgery may not be necessary, as spontaneous recovery may be more common than generally appreciated. 36 refs.

Zervas NT and Mendelson G: Treatment of acute hemorrhage of pituitary tumors. ***Lancet,*** **1:604–605, 1975.**
Three cases of hemorrhage into a pituitary tumor are described with sudden headache, visual loss and mental changes in patients with unsuspected pituitary tumors. Transnasal needle drainage resulted in marked improvement of symptoms. 3 refs.

THYROID DISORDERS

Physiology and Diagnosis

Brown J, Chopra IJ, Cornell JS et al.: Thyroid physiology in health and disease. ***Ann Intern Med,*** **81:68–81, 1974.**
A somewhat specialized review on control of TSH secretion, TSH chemistry, actions of T_4 vs. T_3, Graves' disease and thyroglobulin. 94 refs.

Carlson HE and Hershman JM: The hypothalamic-pituitary-thyroid axis. ***Med Clin North Am,*** **59:1,045–1,053, 1975.**
A brief, clear discussion on the use of TRH testing in thyroid and pituitary disease. 32 refs.

Burger HG and Patel YC: Thyrotropin releasing hormone—TRH. ***Clin Endocrinol Metab,*** **6:83–100, 1977.**
A brief review of TRH physiology and usefulness as a diagnostic test in thyroid and pituitary disease. 68 refs.

Scanlon MF, Rees Smith B and Hall R: Thyroid-stimulating hormones: Neuroregulation and clinical applications. ***Clin Sci Mol Med,*** **55:1–10, 129–138, 1978.**
A complete, recent review of physiology of TSH, and its use in therapy and diagnosis of pituitary and thyroid disorders. 215 refs.

Schimmel M and Utiger RD: Thyroidal and peripheral production of thyroid hormones. Review of recent findings and their clinical implications. *Ann Intern Med,* 87:760–768, 1977.
An excellent review of relationships among T_4, T_3 and reverse T_3 in thyroid and systemic illnesses, with emphasis on diagnostic tests. 94 refs.

Volpe R: The role of autoimmunity in hypoendocrine and hyperendocrine function: With special emphasis on autoimmune thyroid disease. *Ann Intern Med,* 87:86–99, 1977.
A review of current theories of autoimmune involvement in the pathogenesis of certain thyroid disorders, especially Graves' disease and Graves' ophthalmopathy. Other autoimmune endocrinopathies are considered. 120 refs.

Allison AC: Self-tolerance and autoimmunity in the thyroid. *N Engl J Med,* 295:821–827, 1976.
A clearly-written review of immunological aspects of Graves' disease and autoimmune thyroiditis, suggesting that autoantibodies may be involved in the ophthalmopathy, myopathy and pre-tibial myxedema of Graves' disease. 16 refs.

Vagenakis AG and Braverman LE: Thyroid function tests: Which one? *Ann Intern Med,* 84:607–608, 1976.
A very brief but clear review of thyroid function tests and their meaning, including the TRH test. 6 refs.

Larsen PR: Testing thyroid function. *Med Clin North Am,* 59:1,063–1,074, 1975.
This article reviews methods and usefulness of various diagnostic tests in thyroid disease, with a good section on evaluation of thyroid-binding globulin levels. 21 refs.

Wenzel KW: Pharmacological interference with in vitro tests of thyroid function. *Metabolism,* 30:717–732, 1981.
The author reviews the effects of drugs on thyroid function tests, and concludes that diagnosis of thyroid disorders by way of the TRH test is often possible, even when interfering drugs are present. 189 refs.

Melmed, S, Geola FL, Reed, AW et al: A comparison of methods assessing thyroid functon in nonthyroidal illness. *J Clin Endocrinol Metab,* 54:300–306, 1982.
Various tests of thyroid function were used to evaluate 135 patients with thyroid and non-thyroid illnesses and 22 controls. Serum TSH levels were the best way to distinguish between patients with primary hypothyroidism and those with non-thyroidal illness with low T4. 37 refs.

Braverman LE and Vagenakis AG. Adverse effects of iodides on thyroid function. ***Med Clin North Am*, 59:1,075–1,088, 1975.**
An excellent review of this complex subject, with practical information on the Wolff-Chaikoff and Jod-Basedow phenomena. 46 refs.

Hershman JM: Use of thyrotropin-releasing hormone in clinical medicine. ***Med Clin North Am*, 62:313–325, 1978.**
A succinct review of the uses to which this important diagnostic test can be put. 31 refs.

Innerfield R and Hollander CS: Thyroidal complications of pregnancy. ***Med Clin North Am*, 61:67–87, 1977.**
A careful review of this subject emphasizing thyroid function during pregnancy, the effects of maternal hypo- and hyperthyroidism on the fetus and how to treat both. 113 refs.

Vagenakis AG, Braverman LE, Azizi F et al.: Recovery of pituitary thyrotropic function after withdrawal of prolonged thyroid suppression therapy. ***N Engl J Med*, 293:681–684, 1975.**
Seven euthyroid women on long-term thyroid hormone therapy were studied to determine the persistence of pituitary-thyroid suppression. After exogenous thyroxine was discontinued, the TSH (basal and response to TRH) took 2 to 5 weeks to recover, with serum T_4 taking at least 4 weeks. 14 refs.

Hillis WS, Bremner WF, Lawrie TDV and Thompson JA: Systolic time intervals in thyroid disease. ***Clin Endocrinol*, 4:617–624, 1975.**
Systolic time intervals were investigated in 20 hyperthyroid and 15 hypothyroid patients. The former showed shortened pre-ejection period and decreased pre-ejection period/left-ventricular ejection time; the hypothyroid patients showed the opposite. The measurements returned toward normal in treated patients, and were themselves somewhat predictive of thyroid status. 19 refs.

Hypothyroidism

Hall R and Scanlon MF: Hypothyroidism: Clinical features and complications. ***Clin Endocrinol Metab*, 8:29–38, 1979.**
A brief but recent overview of the clinical manifestations of hypothyroidism. 29 refs.

Lamberg BA: Aetiology of hypothyroidism. ***Clin Endocrinol Metab*, 8:3–19, 1979.**
An extremely organized review of most common and uncommon causes of hypothyroidism. About 120 refs.

Watanakunakorn C, Hodges RE and Evans TC: Myxedema: A study of 400 cases. ***Arch Intern Med,*** **116:183–190, 1965.**
A large, classic series of cases of hypothyroidism. Of 400 patients, 83 percent were women. The etiology was classified as ''spontaneous atrophy'' in 43 percent; post-^{131}I in 22 percent; surgery in 17 percent and thyroiditis in 8 percent. The most common symptoms and signs were: (1) dry skin and coarse hair (89 percent); (2) fatigue (70 percent); (3) edema (67 percent); (4) pallor (59 percent); (5) cold intolerance (58 percent) and (6) hoarseness (48 percent). 49 refs.

Bronsky D, Kiamko RT and Waldstein SS: Posttherapeutic myxedema. Relative occurrence after treatment of hyperthyroidism by radioactive iodine (^{131}I) or subtotal thyroidectomy. ***Arch Intern Med,*** **121:113–117, 1968.**
Patients who were hypothyroid after subtotal thyroidectomy (53) or ^{131}I therapy (39) were studied. Patients from both groups developed hypothyroidism at qualitatively similar rates during long-term follow-up, although the incidence of hypothyroidism was somewhat lower in the surgical group. 10 refs.

Schimpff SC, Diggs CH, Wiswell JG et al.: Radiation-related thyroid dysfunction: Implications for the treatment of Hodgkin's disease. ***Ann Intern Med,*** **92: 91–98, 1980.**
Of 169 patients treated with mantle irradiation for Hodgkin's disease, 66 percent had evidence of thyroid dysfunction. This evolved slowly after irradiation. The authors recommend monitoring thyroid function in patients who received mantle irradiation. 32 refs.

Vagenakis AG, Dole K and Braverman LE: Pituitary enlargement, pituitary failure and primary hypothyroidism. ***Ann Intern Med,*** **85:195–198, 1976.**
Two cases of sellar enlargement secondary to long-standing hypothyroidism are described. In these patients, the TSH-secreting pituitary tumor compromised anterior pituitary function. 25 refs.

Onishi T, Miyai K, Aono T et al.: Primary hypothyroidism and galactorrhea. ***Am J Med,*** **63:373–378, 1977.**
Studies in 16 women with primary hypothyroidism revealed that ten had high prolactin levels, 5 of whom had persistent galactorrhea. Correction of hypothyroidism with triiodothyronine normalized prolactin and stopped galactorrhea. The authors postulate that TRH can cause galactorrhea in suceptible patients. 28 refs.

Illig R: Congenital hypothyroidism. ***Clin Endocrinol Metab,*** **8:49–62, 1979.**
A concise discussion of this important topic with emphasis on screening the newborn. 26 refs.

Ridgway EC, McCammon JA, Benotti J and Maloof F: Acute metabolic responses in myxedema to large doses of intravenous L-thyroxine. ***Ann Intern Med,*** **77:549–555, 1972.**
Large doses of intravenous thyroxine (.4 to .75 mg IV, followed by daily injections of .1 to .2 mg) were given to 14 patients with hypothyroidism. A fall in TSH was noted in the first 24 hours; T_4 to T_3 conversion occurred during the first week; but the cortisol response to hypoglycemia remained impaired after 10 days of therapy. 25 refs.

Refetoff S: Thyroid hormone therapy. ***Med Clin North Am,*** **59:1,147–1,162, 1975.**
A practical review of this neglected subject, with emphasis on preparations, dosage and monitoring of hormone therapy for replacement and suppression. 51 refs.

Blum M: Myxedema coma. ***Am J Med Sci,*** **264:432–443, 1972.**
A readable and complete review of this topic, with emphasis on clinical features helpful in differentiating this condition from other causes of coma. Steroid and thyroid therapy are discussed. 72 refs.

Derubertis FR Jr., Michelis MF, Bloom ME et al.: Impaired water excretion in myxedema. ***Am J Med,*** **51:41–53, 1971.**
16 hypothyroid patients and 18 normal subjects underwent a water load test. The hypothyroid patients were found to have impaired free water excretion, apparently related to factors other than inappropriate ADH secretion. The abnormality improved with treatment in 11 patients. 64 refs.

Scarpalezos S, Lygidakis C, Papageorgiou C et al.: Neural and muscular manifestations of hypothyroidism. ***Arch Neurol,*** **29:140–144, 1973.**
Of 51 patients with hypothyroidism, 18 had abnormal electromyograms and 19 had abnormal motor conduction; 30 of 41 had abnormal EEGs. However, findings consistent with myopathy were present in only four patients. 38 refs.

Zwillich CZ, Pierson DJ, Hofeldt FD et al.: Ventilatory control in myxedema and hypothyroidism. ***N Engl J Med,*** **292:662–665, 1975.**
17 hypothyroid patients were studied, and were found to have a blunted respiratory response to hypoxia which improved

with replacement therapy. The authors speculate that this may contribute to the hypoventilation of myxedema. 12 refs.

Bough EW, Crowley WF, Ridgway EC et al.: Myocardial function in hypothyroidism. Relation to disease severity and response to treatment. *Arch Intern Med,* 138:1,476–1,480, 1978.
29 hypothyroid patients had decreased myocardial contractility compared to normal controls, the severity of the cardiac dysfunction correlating roughly with the degree of hypothyroidism. Systolic time intervals normalized after treatment. 25 refs.

Kerber RE and Sherman B: Echocardiographic evaluation of pericardial effusion in myxedema: Incidence and biochemical and clinical correlations. *Circulation,* 52:823–827, 1975.
33 unselected patients with hypothyroidism were studied by echocardiography. 30 percent had pericardial effusions; the patients with effusions had lower heart rates but were not more hypothyroid than patients without effusions. No patients developed tamponade; the effusions cleared with thyroid replacement. 11 refs.

Thyroiditis

Subacute Thyroiditis

Volpé R: Thyroiditis. Current views of pathogenesis. *Med Clin North Am,* 59:1,163–1,175, 1975.
A brief review comparing the clinical and pathological syndromes of DeQuervain's (subacute) and Hashimoto's thyroiditis, with an extensive literature review. 99 refs.

Volpé R: Subacute (DeQuervain's) thyroiditis. *Clin Endocrinol Metab,* 8:81–95, 1979.
An extensive review by one of the prominent authors in the field; his distinction between painless and painful varieties puts him at odds with many current authorities. 80 refs.

Hamburger JI: Subacute thyroiditis: Diagnostic difficulties and simple treatment. *J Nucl Med,* 15:81–89, 1974.
A concise review of the diagnosis and treatment of this syndrome, in which data from 62 patients are reviewed. 28 refs.

Greene JN: Subacute thyroiditis. *Am J Med,* 51:97–108, 1971.
An excellent and complete review of the older literature, with still current recommendations for treatment. The difficulties in differential diagnosis are emphasized. 166 refs.

Ogihara T, Yamamoto T, Azukizawa M et al.: Serum thyrotropin and thyroid hormones in the course of subacute thyroiditis. ***J Clin Endocrinol Metab,*** **37:602–606, 1973.**
Thyroid function tests were followed serially in three patients with subacute thyroiditis. TSH and radioactive iodine uptake were low during the initial hyperthyroid phase; both rose during the subsequent hypothyroid phase. 10 refs.

Hashimoto's Thyroiditis

Doniach D, Bottazzo GF and Russell RCG: Goitrous autoimmune thyroiditis (Hashimoto's disease). ***Clin Endocrinol Metab,*** **8:63–80, 1979.**
A recent, clinically-oriented review of this subject. 65 refs.

Gordin A and Lamberg BA: Natural course of symptomless autoimmune thyroiditis. ***Lancet,*** **2:1,234–1,238, 1975.**
18 patients with Hashimoto's thyroiditis were followed: 28 percent became hypothyroid and 72 percent remained euthyroid up to 28 to 50 months. Those that developed early hypothyroidism had elevated TSH levels and exaggerated responses to TRH at the time of diagnosis. 25 refs.

Fisher DA, Oddie TH, Johnson DE and Nelson JC: The diagnosis of Hashimoto's thyroiditis. ***J Clin Endocrinol Metab,*** **40:795–801, 1975.**
Records from 217 patients with Hashimoto's thyroiditis were reviewed. The authors determined that the diagnosis could be made with high probability if 5 pieces of information were available: physical exam of thyroid; antithyroglobulin antibodies; TSH; radioactive iodine uptake and scan; and the perchlorate discharge test. 11 refs.

Buchanan WW and Harden RM: Primary hypothyroidism and Hashimoto's thyroiditis: A continuous spectrum. ***Arch Intern Med,*** **115:411–417, 1965.**
71 patients with primary hypothyroidism and 50 patients with Hashimoto's disease were studied. Both were much more common in women (8 to 9 : 1) and occurred in middle age, but the Hashimoto's patients had a much higher percentage of positive antithyroid antibody titers (76 percent vs. 16 percent). 46 refs.

Brown J, Solomon DH, Beall GN et al.: Autoimmune thyroid diseases—Graves' and Hashimoto's. ***Ann Intern Med,*** **88:379–391, 1978.**
This report of a UCLA conference reviews the similarities

and differences between these two "autoimmune" disorders, with emphasis on evidence for autoimmunity in patients and families, and some recent evidence on HLA linkage. 80 refs.

Volpé R: The role of autoimmunity in hypoendocrine and hyperendocrine function, with special emphasis on autoimmune thyroid disease. ***Ann Intern Med,*** **87:86–99, 1977.**
A detailed review of autoimmune theories of Graves' disease and Hashimoto's disease, with some interesting speculation on the role of antireceptor antibodies in these conditions. 120 refs.

Papapetrou PD, Lazarus JH, MacSween RMN and Harden RM: Long-term treatment of Hashimoto's thyroiditis with thyroxine. ***Lancet,*** **2:1,045–1,048, 1972.**
12 women with Hashimoto's thyroiditis were followed on thyroxine therapy; 5 were hypothyroid and 7 were euthyroid before therapy, but all of 12 were hypothyroid when therapy was stopped after 10 years. Replacement therapy also decreased goiter size in 11 patients, and seems to be indicated even in euthyroid Hashimoto's. 21 refs.

Spontaneously Resolving Lymphocytic Thyroiditis with Hyperthyroidism

Gluck FB, Nusynowitz ML and Plymate S: Chronic lymphocytic thyroiditis, thyrotoxicosis and low radioactive iodine uptake: Report of four cases. ***N Engl J Med,*** **293:624–628, 1975.**
Four patients are described with transient hyperthyroidism, low radioactive iodide uptake and lymphocytic thyroiditis; these patients appear to have a relatively newly described disease called "spontaneously resolving hyperthyroidism with lymphocytic thyroiditis." 12 refs.

Woolf PD and Daly R: Thyrotoxicosis with painless thyroiditis. ***Am J Med,*** **60:73–79, 1976.**
Five patients with painless, transient hyperthyroidism with low radioactive iodide uptake are described. Sedimentation rate and antithyroid antibodies were normal or minimally increased. These authors consider this a painless form of subacute thyroiditis, with a similar time course. 11 refs.

Dorfman SG, Cooperman MT, Nelson R et al.: Painless thyroiditis and transient hyperthyroidism without goiter. ***Ann Intern Med,*** **86:24–28, 1977.**
Eight more patients with this syndrome are described; all had thyrotoxicosis without goiter, with low radioactive iodide up-

take. Initial levels of antithyroglobulin antibodies were elevated in all patients, in contrast to standard antithyroid antibodies. 18 refs.

Gorman CA, Duick DS, Woolner LB and Wahner HW: Transient hyperthyroidism in patients with lymphocytic thyroiditis. *Mayo Clin Proc,* 53:359–365, 1978.
Four patients with seven episodes of transient, painless hyperthyroidism were studied. All patients had palpable glands, low radioactive iodide uptake and biopsy findings of lymphocytic infiltration; hyperthyroidism resolved spontaneously in 1 to 3 months. 42 refs.

Hyperthyroidism

General and Diagnostic Tests

Kaplan MM and Utiger RD: Diagnosis of hyperthyroidism. *Clin Endocrinol Metab,* 7:97–113, 1978.
A brief overview of diagnostic tests in hyperthyroidism. 44 refs.

Ramsay ID: Muscle dysfunction in hyperthyroidism. *Lancet,* 2:931–935, 1966.
54 consecutive hyperthyroid patients were examined for muscle abnormalities. 50 percent of patients complained of thigh weakness, fewer of proximal arm weakness. Nearly 82 percent had muscle wasting on examination; 93 percent of patients had evidence of myopathy on electromyography; biopsies showed characteristic changes and function returned to normal with treatment. 47 refs.

Smith DA, Fraser SA and Wilson GM: Hyperthyroidism and calcium metabolism. *Clin Endocrinol Metab,* 2:333–354, 1973.
An excellent and complete review of hyperthyroid bone disease and related disorders of calcium metabolism. 50 refs.

Burrow GN: Maternal-fetal considerations in hyperthyroidism. *Clin Endocrinol Metab,* 7:115–125, 1978.
A review of thyroid physiology and the treatment of thyrotoxicosis during pregnancy. The author concludes that the choice between surgery and antithyroid drug therapy is largely an emotional one. 31 refs.

Graves' Disease

Kidd A, Okita N, Row VV and Volpé R: Immunologic aspects of Graves' and Hashimoto's diseases. *Metabolism,* 29: 80–99, 1980.

In the latest of a series of similar reviews, the authors discuss the evidence linking immunologic defects to various thyroid disorders. 155 refs.

Volpé R: The pathogenesis of Graves' disease: An overview. *Clin Endocrinol Metab,* 7:3–29, 1978.
A recent and fairly comprehensive review of the immunologic factors thought to be important in Graves' disease. 139 refs.

Solomon DH, Karen E and Kleeman BA: Concepts of pathogenesis of Graves' disease. *Ann Intern Med,* 22:273–299, 1976.
An interesting review of possible causes of Graves' disease other than the widely held autoimmune theory. 104 refs.

McKenzie JM, Zakarija M and Bonnyus M: Graves' disease. *Med Clin North Am,* 59:1,177–1,192, 1975.
A concise review of the etiology, diagnosis and clinical features of Graves' disease. 65 refs.

Kendall-Taylor P: LATS and human-specific thyroid stimulator: Their relation to Graves' disease. *Clin Endocrinol Metab,* 4:319–339, 1975.
This review is a discussion of what was known about LATS, LATS-protector and human-specific thyroid stimulator in 1975. 70 refs.

Hayles AB, Ed.: Symposium on Graves' disease. *Mayo Clin Proc,* 47:801–995, 1972.
A complete issue is devoted to Graves' disease, with articles on pathogenesis, genetics and some interesting papers on thyroid hormone action on the liver and heart. The lead article is a still current summary of many facets of Graves' disease. 111 refs.

Friedman JM and Fialkow PJ: The genetics of Graves' disease. *Clin Endocrinol Metab,* 7:47–65, 1978.
A review of genetic factors in Graves' disease, describing the high incidence in monozygotic twins (50 percent), the association with the HLA-B8 antigen and the relation to other autoimmune disorders. 132 refs.

Gorman CA: The presentation and management of endocrine ophthalmopathy. *Clin Endocrinol Metab,* 7:67–96, 1978.
A complete review of modern approaches to Graves' ophthalmopathy, with an emphasis on treatment. About 164 refs.

Solomon DH, Chopra IJ, Chopra U et al.: Identification of subgroups of euthyroid Graves' ophthalmopathy. *N Engl J Med,* 296:181–186, 1977.

Of 22 patients with "euthyroid Graves' ophthalmopathy," 6 had characteristics of Graves' and Hashimoto's diseases, 5 had evidence of isolated Graves' ophthalmopathy with no evidence of thyroid disease and 6 could not be classified. This syndrome appears to be heterogeneous rather than simply coexistent with Graves' and Hashimoto's diseases. 39 refs.

Grove AS: Evaluation of exophthalmos. ***N Engl J Med,*** **292:1,005–1,013, 1975.**
An ophthalmologist's view of the diagnostic radiographic evaluation of exophthalmos, primarily of Graves' disease. 91 refs.

Werner SC, Coleman DJ and Franzen LA: Ultrasonographic evidence of a consistent orbital involvement in Graves' disease. ***N Engl J Med,*** **290:1,447–1,450, 1974.**
Of 47 patients with Graves' disease, 30 had no or "non-threatening" eye changes. Ultrasonic evaluation revealed equivocal or no changes in only three patients, suggesting that nearly all patients with Graves' disease have characteristic ocular changes detectable by ultrasound. 12 refs.

Hamburger JI and Sugar HS: What the internist should know about the ophthalmopathy of Graves' disease. ***Arch Intern Med,*** **129:131–139, 1972.**
A readable and well-illustrated review of the basic management of Graves' ophthalmopathy by medical and surgical means. 21 refs.

Werner SC: Classification of the eye changes of Graves' disease. ***J Clin Endocrinol Metab,*** **29:982–984, 1969.**
A brief description of the American Thyroid Association's classification of Graves' ophthalmopathy. No refs.

Treatment

Braverman LE: Therapeutic considerations. ***Clin Endocrinol Metab,*** **7:221–240, 1978.**
The author reviews the kinds of therapy available for several common types of thyrotoxicosis; the treatment of Graves' disease is discussed as an extended example. 88 refs.

Roudebush CP, Hoye KE and DeGroot LJ: Compensated low-dose ^{131}I therapy of Graves' disease. ***Ann Intern Med,*** **87:441–443, 1977.**
The authors treated 62 patients with Graves' disease with a protocol that compensated for the size of the thyroid, rather than with 50 μCi/g as they had done previously. Results after

1 year were: 66 percent euthyroid, 24 percent hyperthyroid and 10 percent hypothyroid. 14 refs.

Safa AM, Schumacher OP and Rodriquez-Antunez A: Long-term follow-up results in children and adolescents treated with radioactive iodine (^{131}I) for hyperthyroidism. ***N Engl J Med,*** **292:167–171, 1975.**
The authors followed 87 children (ages 3 to 18) for a mean of 12.3 years following radioactive iodide therapy for Graves' disease. Hyperthyroidism recurred in 1 patient; hypothyroidism developed in 46 percent and no cancers were noted. 55 refs.

Toft AD, Irvine WJ, Seth J et al.: Thyroid function in long-term follow-up of patients treated with iodine-131 for thyrotoxicosis. ***Lancet,*** **2:576–578, 1975.**
233 euthyroid patients were evaluated who had received ^{131}I for hyperthyroidism 6 to 18 years earlier. Patients with an elevated TSH progressed to hypothyroidism at about 2 to 5 percent per year, whereas patients with normal TSH levels remained euthyroid. 19 refs.

Hayek A, Chapman EM and Crawford JD: Long-term results of treatment of thyrotoxicosis in children and adolescents with radioactive iodine. ***N Engl J Med,*** **283:949–953, 1970.**
30 children (ages 8 to 18) were treated with radioactive iodine for hyperthyroidism, with a mean follow-up period of 9.2 years. No cancers developed; 18 normal children were born to patients. One patient had recurrent hyperthyroidism; permanent hypothyroidism was noted in eight. 34 refs.

Slingerland DW and Burrows BA: Long-term antithyroid treatment in hyperthyroidism. ***JAMA,*** **242:2,408–2,410, 1979.**
Of 80 patients with diffuse toxic goiter and hyperthyroidism given long-term treatment with thioureas (mean: 4.4 years), long-term remissions were achieved in 76 percent. Side effects were rare; two patients developed permanent hypothyroidism. (See also accompanying editorial.) 14 refs.

Gwinup G: Prospective randomized comparison of propylthiouracil. ***JAMA,*** **239:2,457–2,459, 1978.**
Patients with Graves' disease (49) received propylthiouracil in a single daily dose or in 3 divided doses (total 450 mg). 10 patients that did not achieve remission after 10 weeks of single dose therapy did so when given divided doses. 9 refs.

Irvine WJ, Gray RS, Toft AD et al.: Spectrum of thyroid function in patients remaining in remission after antithyroid drug therapy for thyrotoxicosis. ***Lancet,*** **2:179–181, 1977.**

110 patients in remission after antithyroid drug therapy for hyperthyroidism were evaluated. 16 percent in remission for longer than 4 years showed some evidence of thyroid failure, stressing the need for long-term follow-up of these patients. 19 refs.

Greer MA, Kammer H and Bouma DJ: Short-term antithyroid drug therapy for the thyrotoxicosis of Graves' disease. ***N Engl J Med*****, 297:173–176, 1976.**
Patients with untreated (31) or previously treated (9) thyrotoxic Graves' disease were treated with methimazole or propylthiouracil until they became euthyroid, after a mean treatment of 3 to 5 months. About 40 percent of patients remained euthyroid after this therapy; longer treatment with antithyroid drugs may not be necessary in Graves' disease. 22 refs.

Geffner DL, Azukizawa M and Hershman JM: Propylthiouracil blocks extrathyroidal conversion of thyroxine to triiodothyronine and augments thyrotropin secretion in man. ***J Clin Invest*****, 55:224–229, 1975.**
15 studies in 7 athyreotic patients receiving T_4 demonstrated an inhibitory effect of propylthiouracil on peripheral conversion of T_4 to T_3, resulting in increased levels of TSH. 43 refs.

Amrhein JA, Kenny FM and Ross D: Granulocytopenia, lupus-like syndrome and other complications of propylthiouracil therapy. ***J Pediatr*****, 76:54–63, 1970.**
Of 38 patients with hyperthyroidism being treated with propylthiouracil, 10 had one or more episodes of leukopenia (7 of these had granulocytopenia). 1 patient developed a lupus-like syndrome; 10 others developed rash, urticaria, fever or other minor side effects. 16 refs.

Kammer H and Srinivasan K: The use of antithyroid drugs in a single daily dose: Treatment of diffuse toxic goiter. ***JAMA*****, 209:1,325–1,327, 1969.**
Of 41 thyrotoxic patients who became euthyroid on multiple daily doses of propylthiouracil or methimazole, 28 remained euthyroid on a single daily morning dose. This appears to be a reasonable way to administer antithyroid drugs, especially if the hyperthyroidism is mild. 9 refs.

McDevitt DG: Propranolol in treatment of thyrotoxicosis: A review. ***Postgrad Med J*****, 52: suppl. 4,157–162, 1976.**
A short review of propranolol's uses in various types of hyperthyroidism. 48 refs.

Mazaferri EL, Reynolds JC, Young RL et al.: Propranolol as

primary therapy for thyrotoxicosis: Results of a long-term prospective study. ***Arch Intern Med,*** **136:50–56, 1976.**
Of 8 patients with mild hyperthyroidism treated with propranolol only for an average of 8 months, 2 became euthyroid but 6 experienced incomplete control of symptoms and continued to have abnormal systolic time intervals. The authors conclude that propranolol alone is inadequate long-term treatment for hyperthyroidism. 30 refs.

Levey GS: The heart and hyperthyroidism. Use of beta-adrenergic blocking drugs. ***Med Clin North Am,*** **59:1,193–1,201, 1975.**
Of 76 patients 1 to 7 years after subtotal thyroidectomy for hyperthyroidism, 3 were hyperthyroid, 13 hypothyroid and 60 euthyroid. 39 of these 60 had raised TSH levels, lower T_4 levels but normal T_3 levels, suggesting that increased conversion to T_3 was occurring in the euthyroid patients with elevated TSH. 16 refs.

Dillon PT, Babe J, Meloni CR et al.: Reserpine in thyrotoxic crisis. ***N Engl J Med,*** **283:1,020–1,023, 1970.**
The authors treated 7 patients with thyroid storm with intramuscular reserpine in doses of .07 to .3 mg/kg over the first 24 hours. The drug caused marked decreases in heart rate and body temperature, and all patients survived. The authors recommend reserpine as an alternative to propranolol in the management of this condition. 23 refs.

Other Causes

Nelson NC and Becker WF: Thyroid crisis: Diagnosis and treatment. ***Ann Surg,*** **170:263–273, 1969.**
The authors describe 21 cases of thyroid storm out of 2,329 patients with hyperthyroidism. 16 patients died. The precipitating factors, differential diagnosis and possible therapies are discussed. 18 refs.

Mackin JF, Canary JJ and Pittman CS: Thyroid storm and its management. ***N Engl J Med,*** **291:1,396–1,398, 1974.**
A very brief review of thyroid storm. The authors discuss the use of antithyroid drugs, iodine and propranolol in the therapy of this condition. 39 refs.

Studer H, Hunziker HR and Ruchti L: Morphologic and functional substrate of thyrotoxicosis caused by nodular goiters. ***Am J Med,*** **65:227–234, 1978.**
Thyroid glands from 11 patients with multinodular goiters and hyperthyroidism could be divided into 4 histologic types, de-

pending on the anatomic distribution of the autonomous follicles. The type was not predictable by scintiscan. 15 refs.

Miller JM: Plummer's disease. ***Med Clin North Am,*** **59: 1,203–1,266, 1975.**
A complete general review of toxic nodular goiter, with emphasis on treatment strategiess 32 refs.

Cooper DS, Ridgway EC and Maloof F: Unusual types of hyperthyroidism. ***Clin Endocrinol Metab,*** **7:199–220, 1978.**
A concise review of several rare types of hyperthyroidism including TSH secreting tumors, iodine-induced thyrotoxicosis, various types of thyroiditis and others. 154 refs.

Vagenakis AG, Wang CA, Burger A et al.: Iodide-induced thyrotoxicosis in Boston. ***N Engl J Med,*** **287:523–527, 1972.**
Of eight patients with nontoxic goiter living in an iodide-sufficient area, four developed hyperthyroidism when given exogenous iodine. The authors warn about the use of iodine-containing compounds in patients with nontoxic goiter. 24 refs.

Savoie JC, Massin JP, Thomopoulos P et al.: Iodine-induced thyrotoxicosis in apparently normal thyroid glands. ***J Clin Endocrinol Metab,*** **41:685–691, 1975.**
10 patients with no history of thyroid disease developed firm goiters and thyrotoxicosis after taking various iodine compounds for several months. The 24-hour uptake of radioactive iodide was very low; the urinary iodine excretion was high. This may represent a rare variation of the Jod-Basedow phenomenon. 21 refs.

Sterling K, Refetoff S and Selenkow HA: T_3-thyrotoxicosis. ***JAMA,*** **213:571–575, 1970.**
26 cases of thyrotoxicosis with normal T_4 and elevated T_3 are described. The etiologies were toxic multinodular goiter in 12 patients, 7 patients with Graves' disease and 6 with recurrent toxic goiter post-treatment. Symptoms and signs, including ophthalmopathy in Graves' disease, were similar to those found in ordinary thyrotoxicosis. 18 refs.

Mestman JH, Manning PR and Hodgman J: Hyperthyroidism and pregnancy. ***Arch Intern Med,*** **134:434–439, 1974.**
Pregnant hyperthyroid women undergoing 37 pregnancies were divided into 3 groups: untreated; treatment with antithyroid drugs and thyroid replacement; and antithyroid treatment alone. The last group had fewer premature infants. Antithyroid drugs alone appeared to be the treatment of choice during pregnancy. 25 refs.

Gorman CA, Wahner HW and Tauxe WN: Metabolic malingerers: Patients who deliberately induced or perpetuate a hypermetabolic or hypometabolic state. ***Am J Med,*** **48:708–714, 1970.**
Three patients with factitious hyperthyroidism are described. This entity is in the differential diagnosis of hyperthyroidism with low radioactive iodine uptake. 31 refs.

Davis PJ and Davis FB: Hyperthyroidism over the age of 60 years. ***Medicine,*** **53:161–181, 1974.**
A review of the syndrome of "apathetic" hyperthyroidism in which 85 cases are discussed. Most common complaints in these elderly patients were palpitations (42 percent), nervousness (38 percent), weight loss and dyspnea on exertion (both 35 percent) and tiredness and weakness (28 percent). 90 refs.

Kempers RD, Dockerty MB, Hoffman DL and Bartholomew LG: Struma ovarii-ascitic, hyperthyroid and asymptomatic syndromes. ***Ann Intern Med,*** **72:883–893, 1970.**
The authors describe 25 patients with struma ovarii, of which 8 had hyperthyroidism. At least two patients with hyperthyroidism became euthyroid when their thyroid glands were removed. 20 of 25 tumors were teratomas; 5 were malignant. 18 refs.

Tolis G, Bird C, Bertrand G et al.: Pituitary hyperthyroidism: Case report and review of the literature. ***Am J Med,*** **64:177–181, 1978.**
The authors describe a woman with a thyrotropin-secreting pituitary adenoma and hyperthyroidism, which regressed after surgical removal of the adenoma. They review the existing literature on this rare cause of hyperthyroidism. 36 refs.

Thyroid Nodules

Beckers C: Thyroid nodules. ***Clin Endocrinol Metab,*** **8:181–192, 1979.**
A brief review of the workup and therapy of thyroid nodules. 60 refs.

Blum M: Managing the solitary thyroid nodule: The role of needle biopsy (Editorial). ***Ann Intern Med,*** **87:375–377, 1977.**
A cautious editorial reviewing indications and usefulness of needle aspiration and biopsy of thyroid nodules, concluding that these procedures are a supplement to clinical evaluation. 9 refs.

Williams J-S and Lowhagen T: Fine needle aspiration cytology in thyroid disease. ***Clin Endocrinol Metab,*** **10:247–266, 1981.**

In this and the following article, the authors discuss in detail the technique and diagnostic usefulness of this controversial procedure. 16 refs.

Gershengorn MC, McClung MR, Chu EW et al.: Fine-needle aspiration cytology in the preoperative diagnosis of thyroid nodules. *Ann Intern Med*, 87:265–269, 1977.
50 patients with cold nodules were evaluated by fine-needle aspiration. Of 33 patients eventually undergoing surgery, there were 1 false-positive and 1 false-negative aspiration, plus 2 false-negative "suspicious" aspiration. 14 refs.

Thijs LG and Wiener JD: Ultrasonic examination of the thyroid gland. *Am J Med*, 60:96–105, 1976.
The value of ultrasonography in the evaluation of 440 patients with various thyroid disorders is discussed. The main value appears to be in distinguishing between solid and cystic thyroid nodules. 38 refs.

Wright HK, Burrow GN, Spaulding S and Sheahan DG: Current therapy of thyroid nodules. *Surg Clin North Am*, 54:277–288, 1974.
A reasonable approach to the evaluation of thyroid nodules, based on clinical and histologic critera. 2 refs.

Psarras A, Papadapoulos SN, Livadas D et al.: The single thyroid nodule. *Br J Surg*, 59:545–548, 1972.
The authors investigated 2,736 patients with single thyroid nodules seen over a 4 year period. The female to male ratio was seven to one. Excision was performed in 692 cases; carcinoma was present in 12 percent, with an incidence of 12.8 percent in cold nodules, 6.6 percent in warm nodules and 0 percent in hot nodules. 33 refs.

Ferriman D, Hennebry TM and Tassopoulos CN: True thyroid adenoma. *Q J Med*, 41:127–139, 1972.
Of 108 nodules in 138 patients with thyroid adenomas, 20 were hot, 31 functioning and 57 cold. Women outnumbered men in the series six to one. Long-term suppression is discussed. 36 refs.

Miller JM: Hyperthyroidism from the thyroid follicle with autonomous function. *Clin Endocrinol Metab*, 7:177–197, 1978.
A review of both autonomous thyroid nodules and toxic multinodular goiter. 23 refs.

Hamburger JI: Solitary autonomously functioning thyroid lesions: Diagnosis, clinical features and pathogenetic considerations. *Am J Med*, 58:740–748, 1975.

Patients with autonomous thyroid nodules were studied, 140 with nontoxic and 24 with toxic nodules. Women predominated 13 to 1 and 3.8 to 1, respectively. The decision to treat surgically or with ^{131}I is discussed. 52 refs.

Burman KD, Earll JM, Johnson MC and Wartofsky L: Clinical observations on the solitary autonomous thyroid nodule. ***Arch Intern Med,*** **134:915–919, 1974.**
Of 54 patients with autonomous nodules, only 2 were hyperthyroid. 48 patients were followed conservatively for a mean of 24 months; no new cases of hyperthyroidism developed. 8 refs.

Horst W, Rösler H, Schneider C and Labhart A: Three hundred six cases of toxic adenoma: Clinical aspects, findings in radioiodine diagnostics, radiochromatography and histology, results of ^{131}I and surgical treatment. ***J Nucl Med,*** **8:515–528, 1967.**
The authors review the diagnosis and management of toxic adenoma in 306 patients. Radioactive iodide was the preferred treatment, since there is little risk of hypothyroidism. In addition, in 79 patients undergoing operation, no cancer was found. 11 refs.

Gorman CA and Robertson JS: Radiation dose in the selection of ^{131}I or surgical treatment for toxic thyroid adenoma. ***Ann Intern Med,*** **89:85–90, 1978.**
The authors discuss the theoretical basis for radioactive iodide therapy of hot nodules. They recommend surgery for young patients with large nodules. 48 refs.

Nontoxic Goiter

Hennemann G: Nontoxic goitre. ***Clin Endocrinol Metab,*** **8:167–179, 1979.**
A brief, recent review of nontoxic or benign multinodular goiter, with emphasis on the evaluation of possible malignancy and on suppression therapy. 62 refs.

Maloof F, Wang CA and Vickery AL Jr.: Non-toxic goiter—Diffuse or nodular. ***Med Clin North Am,*** **59:1,221–1,232, 1975.**
A brief review of this group of disorders, with emphasis on needle biopsy in diagnosis. 26 refs.

Barsano CP and DeGroot LJ: Dyshormonogenetic goitre. ***Clin Endocrinol Metab,*** **8:145–165, 1979.**
A complete, recent review of these unusual and often familial forms of defective thyroid hormone synthesis. About 132 refs.

Ibbertson HK: Endemic goitre and cretinism. ***Clin Endocrinol Metab,*** **8:97–128, 1979.**
A fascinating and detailed review of these disorders, now relatively uncommon in the United States, but still prevalent in many parts of the world. About 122 refs.

Miller JM and Block MA: Functional autonomy in multinodular goiter. ***JAMA,*** **214:535–539, 1970.**
Of 70 patients with large multinodular goiters, 46 failed to suppress after T_3 administration. The authors caution that this may represent autonomy of thyroid tissue, and that suppression therapy may lead to hyperthyroidism. 5 refs.

Shambaugh GE III, Seed R and Korn A: Airway obstruction in substernal goiter. Clinical and therapeutic implications. ***J Chronic Dis,*** **26:737–743, 1973.**
Five patients with varying degrees of tracheal compression by substernal goiter are described. The authors discuss the evaluation and prevention of this entity. 19 refs.

Dige-Petersen H and Hammer L: Serum thyrotropin concentrations under basal conditions and after stimulation with thyrotropin-releasing hormone in idiopathic non-toxic goiter. ***J Clin Endocrinol Metab,*** **44:1,115–1,120, 1977.**
10 of 37 patients with euthyroid multinodular goiter failed to respond with an adequate TSH rise to TRH stimulation, suggesting thyroid autonomy. 23 refs.

Sokal JE: The problem of malignancy in nodular goiter-recapitulation and a challenge. ***JAMA,*** **170:405–412, 1959.**
The author reviews his earlier data on the subject, and concludes that cancer in multinodular goiters is much more rare than previously thought. 19 refs.

Schimaoka K and Sokal JE: Suppressive therapy of non-toxic goiter. ***Am J Med,*** **57:576–583, 1974.**
Patients with nontoxic goiter (114) were treated with either T_3 or T_4 in a double-blind fashion. 40 of 54 patients treated with T_3 and 29 of 59 patients treated with T_4 showed decreased goiter size in 28 weeks. The authors conclude that T_3 was more effective in shrinking large goiters than T_4. 38 refs.

Thyroid Cancer Excluding Medullary Carcinoma

Thompson NW, Nishiyama RH and Harness JK: Thyroid carcinoma: Current controversies. ***Curr Probl Surg,*** **15(11):1–67, 1978.**

A detailed review of surgical aspects of the management of thyroid carcinoma. 151 refs.

Thomas CG Jr. and Buckwalter JA: Cancer of the thyroid. ***Adv Surg*, 10:245–285, 1976.**
A complete review of these cancers with a somewhat surgical slant. 74 refs.

DeGroot L: Thyroid carcinoma. ***Med Clin North Am*, 59:1,233–1,246, 1975.**
A brief review of the most common types of thyroid cancer, with emphasis on diagnostic and treatment strategies. 30 refs.

Wang CA, Vickery AL Jr. and Maloof F: Needle biopsy of the thyroid. ***Surg Gynecol Obstet*, 143:365–368, 1976.**
Needle biopsies were carried out in 906 patients. 91 biopsies showed no diagnostic abnormality, 725 showed a benign disorder and the remaining 90 patients underwent operation. The preoperative diagnosis was confirmed in 90 percent of cases. One needle track implantation occurred, in which the tumor was a metastatic hypernephroma; there were no operative deaths. 4 refs.

Williams ED: The aetiology of thyroid tumours. ***Clin Endocrinol Metab*, 8:193–207, 1979.**
A concise review of the different types of thyroid cancer, with comments on the epidemiology and etiology of the various kinds. 58 refs.

Roudebush CP, Asteris GT and DeGroot LJ: Natural history of radiation-associated thyroid cancer. ***Arch Intern Med*, 138:1,631–1,634, 1978.**
91 patients with radiation-related thyroid carcinoma were evaluated. 90 percent of the tumors were papillary; there were higher incidences of multicentric, locally invasive and metastatic disease than in autopsy series. 20 refs.

Favus MJ, Schneider AB, Stachura ME et al.: Thyroid cancer occurring as a late consequence of head and neck irradiation. ***N Engl J Med*, 294:1,019–1,025, 1976.**
1,056 patients were examined who had received head and neck irradiation between 1939 and 1962 for benign disease. 16.5 percent had palpable thyroid nodules, with an additional 10.7 percent having nodules on scintiscan (overall prevalence: 27.2 percent). 60 of 182 patients with nodules operated on had thyroid cancer, which is thus a risk after childhood irradiation. 25 refs.

Hempleman LH, Hall WJ, Phillips M et al.: Neoplasms in persons treated with x-rays in infancy: Fourth survey in 20 years. ***J Natl Cancer Inst,*** **55:519–530, 1975.**
This was the fourth survey of thyroid cancers in 2,872 patients who received neck irradiation in infancy. The overall risk of developing cancer was 2.5 per year per million people per rad; the risk was higher in young women and Jews. 24 refs.

Arnold J, Pinsky S, Ryo UY et al.: ^{99m}Tc-pertechnetate thyroid scintigraphy in patients predisposed to thyroid neoplasms by prior radiotherapy to the head and neck. ***Radiology,*** **115:653–657, 1975.**
Thyroid scans were performed in 1,452 patients with a previous history of neck irradiation. Abnormal scans were obtained in 21 percent; cancer was found in 29 percent of the 193 patients who underwent surgery. Of the cancers, 96 percent were noted on scan. 19 refs.

Dobyns BM, Sheline GE, Workman JB et al.: Malignant and benign neoplasms of the thyroid in patients treated for hyperthyroidism: A report of the cooperative thyrotoxicosis follow-up study. ***J Clin Endocrinol Metab,*** **38:976–998, 1974.**
This multicenter trial followed 36,050 patients after treatment for hyperthyroidism. The risk of thyroid cancer was not increased in patients receiving ^{131}I therapy compared to other treatment modalities. 51 refs.

Holm LE, Dahlquist I, Israelsson A and Lundell G: Malignant thyroid tumors after iodine-131 therapy. A retrospective cohort study. ***N Engl J Med,*** **303:188–191, 1980.**
The incidence of thyroid tumors in 3,000 patients treated with radioactive iodine (2,727 for hyperthyroidism and 273 for cardiac disease) was no different from the incidence expected in the general population. Mean follow-up was 13 years for the hyperthyroid patients and 6 years for the cardiac patients (see accompanying editorial). 29 refs.

Halnan KE: The influence of age and sex on incidence and prognosis of thyroid cancer: 344 cases followed for ten years. ***Cancer,*** **19:1534–1542, 1966.**
Survival data were accumulated on 344 patients with thyroid cancer presenting to one hospital between 1945 and 1955. Prognosis became poorer with increasing age at diagnosis. 4 refs.

Edmonds CJ: Treatment of thyroid cancer. ***Clin Endocrinol Metab,*** **8:223–242, 1979.**
A general review of thyroid cancer, with specific comments

on medullary, follicular and anaplastic carcinomas. About 70 refs.

Sanfelippo PM, Beahrs AH, McConahey WM et al.: Indications for thyroidectomy. ***Mayo Clin Proc,*** **48:269–272, 1973.**
Of 3,000 patients with goiter seen at the Mayo Clinic over 1 year, 365 underwent thyroidectomy, mainly for nodular goiter. Of these patients, one suffered damage to the recurrent laryngeal nerve, and three developed permanent hypoparathyroidism. 17 refs.

Block MA: Management of carcinoma of the thyroid. ***Ann Surg,*** **185:133–144, 1977.**
A review of the various surgical approaches to different histologic types and extents of thyroid cancer. Prognostic factors are discussed. 103 refs.

Thompson NW and Harness JK: Complications of total thyroidectomy for carcinoma. ***Surg Gynecol Obstet,*** **131:861–868, 1970.**
This sobering paper discusses the surgical complications of 184 total thyroidectomies for cancer. Unilateral single recurrent laryngeal nerve damage occurred in 12 percent; hypocalcemia occurred in 22 percent, with permanent hypoparathyroidism in 5.4 percent. There were no operative deaths. 8 refs.

Mazzaferri EL, Young RL, Oertel JE et al.: Papillary thyroid carcinoma: The impact of therapy in 576 patients. ***Medicine,*** **56:117–123, 1977.**
This review discussed 576 patients with papillary carcinoma treated at various centers. The authors concluded that thyroxine therapy is indicated in all patients, that total thyroidectomy is indicated for lesions larger than 2.5 cm, and ablative ^{131}I therapy should be employed postoperatively in most cases. 123 refs.

Thomas CG: Surgery of the thyroid. ***Med Clin North Am,*** **59:1247–1261, 1975.**
A review of surgical treatment of thyrotoxicosis and thyroid cancer. 24 refs.

Busnardo B, Vangelista R, Girelli ME et al.: TSH levels and TSH response to TRH as a guide to the replacement treatment of patients with thyroid carcinoma. ***J Clin Endocrinol Metab,*** **42:901–906, 1976.**
46 patients with thyroid carcinoma were treated with T_3 following thyroid ablation. In some patients whose TSH levels

were brought within normal limits, the response to TRH was exaggerated; increasing the dose of T_3 prevented this response. 14 refs.

Charles MA, Dodson LE Jr., Waldeck N et al.: Serum thyroglobulin levels predict total body iodine scan findings in patients with treated, well-differentiated thyroid carcinoma. ***Am J Med,*** **69:401–407, 1980.**
Of 48 patients with treated, well-differentiated thyroid carcinoma, 24 had both normal ^{131}I body scans and serum thyroglobulin levels. In contrast, thyroglobulin levels were elevated in eight patients with metastatic disease, suggesting that this may be a useful marker of disease recurrence in these patients. 23 refs.

Medullary Carcinoma

Chong GC, Beahrs OH, Sizemore GW and Woolner LH: Medullary carcinoma of the thyroid gland. ***Cancer,*** **35:695–704, 1975.**
The authors evaluated almost 50 years of experience with medullary cancer at the Mayo Clinic, comprising 139 patients. The tumor represented 8 percent of all thyroid cancers; 21 percent occurred in patients with either MEN 2a or 2b; and the 5 and 10 year survival rates after surgey were 80 percent and 67 percent, respectively. 33 refs.

Hill CS Jr., Ibanez ML, Samaan NA et al.: Medullary (solid) carcinoma of the thyroid gland: An analysis of the M.D. Anderson Hospital experience with patients with the tumor, its special features and its histogenesis. ***Medicine,*** **52:141–171, 1973.**
A review of the syndrome as seen at one hospital, comprising 73 patients (9 percent of patients with thyroid cancer). Calcitonin was invariably elevated in serum; 32 percent of patients experienced severe diarrhea; several instances of ectopic ACTH production were noted; 5 year survival was 72 percent of all patients. 95 refs.

Graze K, Spiler IJ, Tashjian AH Jr. et al.: Natural history of familial medullary thyroid carcinoma. Effect of a program for early diagnosis. ***N Engl J Med,*** **299:980–985, 1978.**
Calcium and/or pentagastrin stimuli of calcitonin secretion were applied yearly to a familial cohort of 107 patients at risk for developing medullary thyroid carcinoma. 21 patients converted to abnormal responses in 7 years; 8 of 21 glands removed showed foci of nonmetastatic carcinoma, arguing for

routine screening to detect early cases of medullary thyroid cancer. 26 refs.

Melvin KEW, Tashjian AH Jr and Miller HH: Studies in familial (medullary) thyroid carcinoma. ***Recent Prog Horm Res,*** **28:399–470, 1972.**
A long and complex review of this tumor, with special reference to studies of calcitonin dynamics in familial varieties of medullary carcinoma. About 93 refs.

Sizemore GW and Go VLW: Stimulation tests for diagnosis of medullary thyroid carcinoma. ***Mayo Clin Proc,*** **50:53–56, 1975.**
These authors compare stimulation of calcitonin by pentagastrin, calcium and glucagon in four patients at high risk for medullary carcinoma. Pentagastrin provided the greatest stimulus in these patients; the methods for conducting all three test are described. 14 refs.

Jackson CE, Tashjian AH Jr. and Block MA: Detection of medullary thyroid cancer by calcitonin assay in families. ***Ann Intern Med,*** **78:845–857, 1973.**
Stimulatory testing with calcitonin measurements was carried out in 76 relatives of patients with medullary carcinoma. 17 of 22 patients with positive tests had surgery, and 16 had cancer. Six patients with positive stimulation tests had normal basal calcitonin concentrations. 23 refs.

Hellman DE, Kartchner M, Van Antwerp JD et al.: Radioiodine in the treatment of medullary carcinoma of the thyroid. ***J Clin Endocrinol Metab,*** **48:451–455, 1979.**
An interesting case report in which residual medullary carcinoma was treated with radioactive iodine after thyroidectomy. The tumor tissue did not take up iodine; however, it appeared sensitive to the high levels of radiation emanating from neighboring thyroid tissue. 32 refs.

ADRENAL DISORDERS

Physiology and Diagnosis

Ganong WF, Alpert LC and Lee TC: ACTH and the regulation of adrenocortical secretion. ***N Engl J Med,*** **290:1,006–1,011, 1974.**
A brief review of ACTH secretion and its effects on the adrenal gland. 9 refs.

Tyler FH and West CD: Laboratory evaluation of disorders of the adrenal cortex. ***Am J Med,*** **53:664–672, 1972.**

A brief review of laboratory aids to the diagnosis of adrenal disease, with specific comments on their applicability in Addison's disease, hypopituitarism, steroid therapy, Cushing's syndrome and congenital adrenal hyperplasia. 25 refs.

Gwinup G and Johnson B: Clinical testing of the hypothalamic-pituitary-adrenocortical system in states of hypo- and hyper-cortisolism. *Metabolism,* 24:777–791, 1975.
A practical review of pituitary-adrenal function testing in Addison's and Cushing's diseases. 87 refs.

Steinbeck AW and Theile HM: The adrenal cortex (excluding aldosteronism). *Clin Endocrinol Metab,* 3:557–591, 1974.
A readable review of adrenal physiology, the laboratory evaluation of adrenal disorders, and the clinical aspects of Cushing's and Addison's diseases and the adrenogenital syndromes. 102 refs.

Burke CW: Hormones in urine: Uses and misuses. *J R Coll Physicians Lond,* 8:335–354, 1974.
A nice review of urinary hormone determinations and their uses, which centers on steroid hormone and metabolite measurements in adrenal and gonadal disorders. 52 refs.

Thompson EB and Lippman ME: Mechanism of action of glucocorticoids. *Metabolism,* 23:159–202, 1974.
An extensive review of what is known about the actions of steroid hormones at the molecular level as well as about physiologic and pharmacologic actions. 352 refs.

Cryer PE: Physiology and pathophysiology of the human sympathoadrenal neuroendocrine system. *N Engl J Med,* 303:436–444, 1980.
A recent review of sympathoadrenal physiology and pathophysiology. 68 refs.

Axelrod S and Weinshilboum R: Catecholamines. *N Engl J Med,* 287:237–242, 1972.
A brief review of catecholamine physiology and pharmacology, with comments on pheochromocytoma. 5 refs.

Thorn GW and Lauler DP: Clinical therapeutics of adrenal disorders. *Am J Med,* 53:673–684, 1972.
A review of the therapeutic management of common adrenal disorders, with special reference to Cushing's syndrome. 4 refs.

Horton R: Aldosterone: Review of its physiology and diagnostic aspects of primary aldosteronism. *Metabolism,* 22:1525–1545, 1973.

The author reviews what was then known about aldosterone physiology and the diagnosis and clinical features of hyperaldosteronism. 176 refs.

Brown JJ, Fraser R, Lever AF and Robertson JIS: Aldosterone: Physiological and pathophysiological variations in man. ***Clin Endocrinol Metab,*** **1:397–449, 1972.**
A long, detailed review of aldosterone physiology and control, and the clinical syndromes associated with abnormal secretion of aldosterone. About 286 refs.

Chan L and O'Malley BW: Steroid hormone action: Recent advances. ***Ann Intern Med,*** **89:694–701, 1978.**
A review of the authors' work on molecular basis for steroid hormone action. 66 refs.

Kehlet H, Blichert-Toft M, Hancke S et al.: Comparative study of ultrasound, ^{131}I-19-iodocholesterol scintigraphy and aortography in localizing adrenal lesions. ***Br Med J,*** **2:665–667, 1976.**
The authors evaluated 27 patients with adrenal disorders who underwent ultrasound, arteriography and adrenal scanning preoperatively. Ultrasound predicted 100 percent of positive findings and 79 percent of negative ones; corresponding values for arteriography were 83 percent and 64 percent, and for adrenal scan were 100 percent and 85 percent. 16 refs.

Addison's Disease

Irvine WJ and Barnes EW: Adrenocortical insufficiency. ***Clin Endocrinol Metab,*** **1:549–594, 1972.**
A complete and detailed review of Addison's disease, with sections on etiology, clinical features, diagnostic tests and a detailed review of immunologic considerations. 57 refs.

Nerup J: Addison's disease—Clinical studies: A report of 108 cases. ***Acta Endocrinol,*** **76:127–141, 1974.**
The author reviewed 108 cases of Addison's disease, diagnosed in Denmark between 1950 and 1972. Etiologies were idiopathic (66 percent), tuberculous (17 percent) or unknown (17 percent). Of patients with the idiopathic variety, 53 percent had associated autoimmune disorders. The clinical features of the syndrome are reviewed. 37 refs.

Tzagournis M: Acute adrenal insufficiency. ***Heart Lung,*** **7:603–609, 1978.**
A brief review of Addison's disease and Addisonian crisis. 11 refs.

Hubay CA, Weckesser EC and Levy RP: Occult adrenal insufficiency in surgical patients. ***Ann Surg,*** **181:325–332, 1975.**
The authors described eight patients who presented with surgical problems and related, occult adrenal insufficiency. They discuss the diagnosis, management and etiologies of this condition in surgical patients. 30 refs.

Speckart PF, Nicoloff JT and Bethune JC: Screening for adrenocortical insufficiency with cosyntropin (synthetic ACTH). ***Arch Intern Med,*** **128:761–763, 1971.**
In a brief but important paper, the authors describe what has become a very important screening test for adrenal insufficiency. 12 refs.

Clark OH, Hall AD and Schambelan M: Clinical manifestations of adrenal hemorrhage. ***Am J Surg,*** **128:219–224, 1974.**
Of 34 patients with adrenal hemorrhage, 32 died. Only 7 of 34 had symptoms clearly related to adrenal hemorrhage; these were prostration, fever, mental abnormalities, vomiting and weakness with severe, constant, localized abdominal pain. It appeared more common in certain clinical scenarios, e.g., in postpartum women or anticoagulated patients. 37 refs.

Wuepper KD, Wegienka LC and Fudenberg HH: Immunologic aspects of adrenocortical insufficiency. ***Am J Med,*** **46:206–216, 1969.**
Antibodies to adrenal tissue were present in serum from 14 of 22 patients with idiopathic Addison's disease; they were not detected in adrenal insufficiency resulting from infection. The patients and relatives had high incidences of other autoantibodies in their sera. 39 refs.

Eisenbarth GS, Wilson PW, Ward F et al.: The polyglandular failure syndrome: Disease inheritance, HLA type and immune function. ***Ann Intern Med,*** **91:528–533, 1979.**
11 patients with "polyglandular failure syndrome" are described. This syndrome appeared to be associated with HLA-B8, and a high incidence was noted among 42 relatives of the original cohort. 40 refs.

Frey HMM, Vogt JH and Nerup J: Familial polyendocrinopathy. ***Acta Endocrinol,*** **72:401–416, 1973.**
Two families with a high incidence of autoimmune endocrinopathies are described. The authors conclude that patients from these families shared a genetic deficiency in immune function, and they review the literature on this syndrome. 84 refs.

Irvine WJ and Barnes EW: Addison's disease, ovarian failure and hypoparathyroidism. ***Clin Endocrinol Metab,*** **4:379–434, 1975.**
The authors review clinical and immunologic aspects of these three conditions, taken separately and together in the "polyglandular failure syndrome." 112 refs.

Carpenter CCJ, Solomon N, Silverberg SG et al.: Schmidt's syndrome (thyroid and adrenal insufficiency): A review of the literature and a report of 15 new cases including ten instances of coexistent diabetes mellitus. ***Medicine,*** **43:153–180, 1964.**
A review of Schmidt's syndrome, in which the authors review the literature and present 15 new cases. Of the new cases, 10 also had diabetes, and many had autoantibodies against thyroid and adrenal tissue. 145 refs.

Schaumburg HH, Powers JM, Raine CS et al.: Adrenoleukodystrophy. A clinical and pathological study of 17 cases. ***Arch Neurol,*** **32:577–591, 1975.**
The authors describe 17 male patients with pathological findings of adrenoleukodystrophy. Patients had clinical and laboratory evidence of primary adrenal failure, but generally more severe neurologic dysfunction; this was due to degeneration of white matter. Open adrenal biopsy was the best diagnostic test. 43 refs.

Griffin JW, Goren E, Schaumburg H et al.: Adrenomyeloneuropathy: A probable variant of adrenoleukodystrophy. ***Neurology,*** **27:1,107–1,113, 1977.**
Four male patients are described with adrenal insufficiency, hypogonadism, spastic paraparesis and other neurologic findings; the disorder appeared to be familial. The authors feel that this is a distinct variant of adrenoleukodystrophy. 18 refs.

Cushing's Syndrome

General

Gold EM: The Cushing syndromes: Changing views of diagnosis and treatment. ***Ann Intern Med,*** **90:829–844, 1979.**
A complete, recent and detailed review of the several diseases making up the Cushing's syndromes. 234 refs.

Besser GM and Edwards CRW: Cushing's syndrome. ***Clin Endocrinol Metab,*** **1:451–490, 1972.**
A detailed, clinically oriented review of Cushing's syndrome and its various causes. 65 refs.

Burke CW and Beardwell CG: Cushing's syndrome: An evaluation of the clinical usefulness of urinary free cortisol and other urinary steroid measurements in diagnosis. ***Q J Med,*** **42:175–204, 1973.**
The authors measured urinary free cortisol levels in response to dexamethazone and metyrapone in 40 patients with Cushing's syndrome and in 34 suspected but later disproved patients. There was no overlap between patients' and controls' 24-hour basal urinary free cortisol excretion, whereas there was with 17-hydroxysteroid levels. They review other available diagnostic tests. 60 refs.

Crapo L: Cushing's syndrome: A review of diagnostic tests. ***Metabolism,*** **28:955–977, 1979.**
A thorough recent review of modern diagnostic approaches to Cushing's syndrome. 222 refs.

Raux MC, Binoux M, Luton JP et al.: Studies of ACTH secretion control in 116 cases of Cushing's syndrome. ***J Clin Endocrinol Metab,*** **40:186–197, 1975.**
The authors measured ACTH levels in 116 patients with Cushing's syndrome. It was low in patients with adrenal tumors (10 patients), high in ectopic ACTH (10) and elevated in Cushing's disease (43). Six patients with nodular adrenal hyperplasia had undetectable levels before treatment. 44 refs.

Hankin ME, Theile HM and Steinbeck AW: An evaluation of laboratory tests for the detection and differential diagnosis of Cushing's syndrome. ***Clin Endocrinol,*** **6:185–196, 1977.**
The authors evaluated diagnostic tests in 25 patients with confirmed Cushing's syndrome. They concluded that urinary free cortisol excretion and diurnal plasma cortisol variation were the most specific, but that normal values may occur with these tests, too. 40 refs.

Eddy RL, Lloyd Jones A, Gilliland PF et al.: Cushing's syndrome: A prospective study of diagnostic methods. ***Am J Med,*** **55:621–630, 1973.**
Of 39 patients with clinical features of Cushing's syndrome and at least 1 elevated plasma cortisol measurement, 24 were proven to have Cushing's syndrome. Urinary free cortisol was elevated in all patients with Cushing's syndrome and was not totally suppressible; all of the other patients suppressed normally. 57 refs.

Schambelan M, Slaton PE Jr. and Biglieri EG: Mineralocorticoid production in hyperadrenocorticism. Role in pathogenesis of hypokalemic alkalosis. ***Am J Med,*** **51:299–303, 1971.**

The authors evaluated seven patients with ectopic ACTH syndrome and 17-hydroxylase deficiency. They had elevated plasma levels of desoxycorticosterone (DOC) and corticosterone, but normal or low aldosterone secretion; cortisol secretion was elevated in the first group but not in the second. The authors attribute the hypokalemic alkalosis of Cushing's to DOC and corticosterone. 25 refs.

Orth DN and Liddle GW: Results of treatment in 108 patients with Cushing's syndrome. *N Engl J Med,* 285:243–247, 1971.
The authors treated 108 patients with Cushing's syndrome (17 had adrenal adenoma, 17 ectopic ACTH, 10 adrenal carcinoma, and 64 Cushing's disease). They discuss the results of therapy specific for each of the various causes of the syndrome. 19 refs.

Aloia JF, Roginsky M, Ellis K et al.: Skeletal metabolism and body composition in Cushing's syndrome. *J Clin Endocrinol Metab,* 39:981–985, 1974.
Total body calcium was decreased in five of seven patients with Cushing's syndrome, as measured by neutron activation analysis and whole body counting. The osteopenia was generally not corrected by treatment of the Cushing's syndrome. 26 refs.

Cushing's Disease (See Also Nelson's Syndrome)

Rovit RL and Duane TD: Cushing's syndrome and pituitary tumors. Pathophysiology and ocular manifestations of ACTH-secreting pituitary adenomas. *Am J Med,* 46:416–426, 1969.
A review of Cushing's disease and the anatomic relationships important in the management of the often aggressive chromophobe adenomas involved. 65 refs.

Urbanic RC and George JM: Cushing's disease—18 years' experience. *Medicine,* 60:14–24, 1981.
The authors evaluated retrospectively 31 patients with Cushing's disease seen at a single institution. They review the symptoms and signs present in these patients as well as diagnostic testing. Of 27 patients treated with bilateral adrenalectomy, 22% developed proven and 22% suspected Nelson's syndrome. 83 refs.

Salassa RM, Laws ER Jr., Carpenter PC and Northcutt RC: Transsphenoidal removal of pituitary microadenoma in Cushing's disease. *Mayo Clin Proc,* 53:24–28, 1978.
18 of 22 patients with endocrinologic evidence of Cushing's

disease underwent transsphenoidal exploration. Clinical remissions occurred in 16 patients, but Cushing's disease persisted in 2 patients. Several patients studied 6 months postoperatively had otherwise normal pituitary function; longer-term follow-up was not described. 24 refs.

Tyrrell JB, Brooks RM, Fitzgerald PA et al.: Selective transsphenoidal resection of pituitary microadenomas. ***N Engl J Med,*** **298:753–758, 1978.**
The authors explored the sellas of 20 patients with Cushing's disease, 8 of whom had normal sellar tomographs. They removed 17 adenomas and 1 whole pituitary; transient diabetes insipidus occurred in 5 patients, and most patients required replacement glucocorticoid therapy. Cushing's syndrome was corrected in 17 patients, but follow-up was short (2 to 6 months). 27 refs.

Orth DN: Metyrapone is useful only as adjunctive therapy in Cushing's disease. ***Ann Intern Med,*** **89:128–130, 1978.**
A brief editorial in which the author describes the appropriate uses of metyrapone in Cushing's disease, of which long-term management is not one. 13 refs.

Jennings AS, Liddle GW and Orth DN: Results of treating childhood Cushing's disease with pituitary irradiation. ***N Engl J Med,*** **297:957–962, 1977.**
15 patients treated in childhood with conventional megavoltage pituitary irradiation for Cushing's disease were evaluated. 12 were cured; 3 patients required bilateral adrenalectomy. No patients were panhypopituitary. 38 refs.

Krieger DT, Amorosa L and Linick F: Cyproheptadine-induced remission of Cushing's disease. ***N Engl J Med,*** **293:893–896, 1975.**
Three patients with Cushing's disease were treated with the antiserotonergic drug, cyproheptadine. All three patients had clinical and laboratory evidence of remission; in one patient, hypercortisolism returned when the drug was stopped. Side effects were apparently minimal. 27 refs.

Luton JP, Mahondeau JA, Bouchard P et al.: Treatment of Cushing's disease by o,p'DDD: Survey of 62 cases. ***N Engl J Med,*** **300:459–464, 1979.**
Of 62 patients with Cushing's disease, 16 received pituitary irradiation and o,p'DDD, and 46 received o,p'DDD alone. Most patients achieved remissions of hypercortisolism with o,p'DDD, although 60 percent relapsed when the drug was stopped. The authors maintain that o,p'DDD with or without

radiation may be appropriate therapy in some cases of Cushing's disease. 29 refs.

Schteingart DE, Tsao HS, Taylor CI et al.: Sustained remission of Cushing's disease with mitotane and pituitary irradiation. *Ann Intern Med*, 92:613–619, 1980.
Of 36 patients with Cushing's disease treated with both pituitary irradiation and mitotane (o,p′DDD), early biochemical improvement was observed in at least 17. Side effects of mitotane included anorexia, nausea, decreased memory and gynecomastia. 29 refs.

Adrenal Cushing's Syndrome and Adrenocortical Carcinoma

Meador CK, Bowdoin B, Owen WC Jr. and Farmer TA Jr.: Primary adrenocortical nodular dysplasia: A rare cause of Cushing's syndrome. *J Clin Endocrinol Metab*, 27:1,255–1,263, 1967.
A controversial case report of bilateral "autonomous" adrenocortical nodular hyperplasia, in a 14 year old girl with Cushing's syndrome. ACTH was undetectable preoperatively, and returned to normal three months postoperatively. Both adrenals contained many small nodules and adrenal tissue. 27 refs.

Ruder HJ, Loriaux DL and Lipsett MB: Severe osteopenia in young adults associated with Cushing's syndrome due to micronodular adrenal disease. *J Clin Endocrinol Metab*, 39:1,138–1,147, 1974.
Two patients with severe osteopenia and minor other findings of Cushing's syndrome are described. ACTH was not detectable in either patient. The adrenals showed micronodular hyperplasia on pathology. The authors review an additional 10 cases of this rare cause of Cushing's syndrome. 20 refs.

Child DF, Burke CW, Burley DM et al.: Drug control of Cushing's syndrome: Combined aminoglutethimide and metyrapone therapy. *Acta Endocrinol*, 82:330–341, 1976.
The authors describe the use of both aminoglutethimide (500 to 750 mg/day) and metyrapone (2 g/day) in the management of 18 patients with Cushing's syndrome of varying etiologies. Clinical and chemical improvement occurred in many patients, who tolerated the combination better than higher dose aminoglutethimide. 20 refs.

Smilo RP, Earll JM and Forsham PH: Suppression of tumorous adrenal hyperfunction by aminoglutethimide. *Metabolism*, 16:374–377, 1967.

6 patients with Cushing's syndrome were treated with aminoglutethimide (1 to 1.5 g/day). Three patients with adrenal tumors responded, but three with Cushing's disease did not. Side effects were reported as minimal. 13 refs.

Scott WH Jr., Foster JH, Rhamy RK et al.: Surgical management of adrenocortical tumors with Cushing's syndrome. *Ann Surg*, 173:892–905, 1971.
The authors describe 28 patients with Cushing's syndrome due to adrenocortical tumors (of 110 patients with Cushing's syndrome). Of the 28, 18 patients had benign adenomata, bilateral in one; 10 patients had adrenocortical carcinoma. The surgical management of these patients is discussed. 18 refs.

Lipsett MB, Hertz R and Ross GT: Clinical and pathophysiologic aspects of adrenocortical carcinoma. *Am J Med*, 35:374–383, 1963.
The authors reviewed 38 patients with adrenocortical carcinoma, as well as many other cases from the literature. The male/female ratio was .17 in patients with Cushing's syndrome and 1.8 in patients without. Of 194 patients, 53 percent had Cushing's syndrome and 3 percent had virilism alone. Almost all patients had high urinary 17-ketosteroid excretion. 28 refs.

Hutter AM Jr. and Kayhoe DE: Adrenal cortical carcinoma. Clinical features of 138 patients. *Am J Med*, 41:572–580, 1966.
Of 138 patients with adrenal cortical carcinoma, 68 percent were female and the mean age was 38. Cushing's syndrome was present in 59 percent, virilization alone in 19 percent and both in 4 percent; an additional 12 percent were feminized, all men, in which gynecomastia was the predominant feature. Urinary 17-ketosteroid excretion was increased in 67 percent. 30 refs.

Hutter AM Jr. and Kayhoe DE: Adrenal cortical carcinoma. Results of treatment with o,p'DDD in 138 patients. *Am J Med*, 41:587–592, 1966.
Of 138 patients with adrenal cortical carcinoma treated with o,p'DDD, 83 percent developed gastrointestinal disturbances, 41 percent neuromuscular disturbances and 14 percent rash. Of 62 patients with high steroid excretion pretreatment, 69 percent had a good steroid response to therapy. 34 percent of patients were reported to have a clinical response. 27 refs.

Temple TE and Liddle GW: Inhibitors of the adrenal steroid biosynthesis. *Ann Rev Pharmacol*, 10:199–215, 1970.

A brief review (one of very few available) of the sites of action, and diagnostic and therapeutic uses of inhibitors of adrenal steroid biosynthesis. 122 refs.

Lubitz JA, Freeman L and Okun R: Mitotane use in inoperable adrenal cortical carcinoma. *JAMA*, 223:1,109–1,112, 1973.
Of 115 patients with inoperable adrenal carcinoma, 85 percent of 61 patients with elevated steroid excretion showed a decrease in this excretion by greater than 30 percent, and 61 percent of 75 patients had a measurable decrease in tumor size. Side effects were gastrointestinal (74 percent), neuromuscular (60 percent), skin (13 percent) and miscellaneous (21 percent). 9 refs.

The Ectopic ACTH Syndrome (See Also Ectopic Hormone Production [General])

Liddle GW, Givens JR, Nicholson WE et al.: The ectopic ACTH syndrome. *Cancer Res*, 25:1,057–1,061, 1965.
A brief review of this syndrome, in which 37 new cases are described. Of the 37, 34 patients died within 6 years of onset of symptoms. 18 refs.

O'Riordan JLH, Blanshard GP, Moxham A and Nabarro JDN: Corticotropin-secreting carcinomas. *Q J Med*, 35:137–147, 1966.
The authors describe 5 new cases of the ectopic ACTH syndrome and review a total of 118 from the literature. Of these cases, 53 percent were associated with oat-cell carcinoma, 12 percent with thymoma and 9 percent with both mediastinal carcinoma and islet-cell carcinoma of the pancreas. 37 refs.

Azzopardi JC and Williams ED: Pathology of "non-endocrine" tumors associated with Cushing's syndrome. *Cancer*, 22:274–286, 1968.
The authors review the literature on the ectopic ACTH syndrome and conclude that ACTH-secreting tumors fall in four main categories: oat-cell carcinoma, foregut endocrine tumors, pheochromocytoma and ovarian tumors. 73 refs.

Imura H, Matsakura S, Yamamoto H et al.: Studies on ectopic ACTH-producing tumors: II. Clinical and biochemical features of 30 cases. *Cancer*, 35:1,430–1,436, 1975.
The authors review 30 cases of ectopic ACTH-producing tumors established by measuring ACTH content of the tumor tissue. 7 of 30 patients did not have Cushing's syndrome.

Many tumors contained other polypeptide hormone activity as well. 29 refs.

Ratcliffe JG, Knight RA, Besser GM et al.: Tumour and plasma ACTH concentrations in patients with and without the ectopic ACTH syndrome. *Clin Endocrinol,* 1:27–44, 1972.
17 tumors from patients with the ectopic ACTH syndrome were compared with 14 tumors from non-Cushingoid patients. Both tumor and serum ACTH levels were elevated in the Cushing's patients, but the tumor levels overlapped somewhat with those from the control tumors, which in turn were higher than in normal tissue. 38 refs.

Congenital Adrenal Hyperplasia (See Also Hirsutism and Virilism [General])

Migeon CJ: Adrenal androgens in man. *Am J Med,* 53:607–626, 1972.
A complete general review of adrenal androgens in man, their measurement in serum and urine and their role in several pathologic conditions, particularly congenital adrenal hyperplasia. 90 refs.

Kaplan SA: Diseases of the adrenal cortex. II. Congenital adrenal hyperplasia. *Pediatr Clin North Am,* 26:77–89, 1979.
A recent review of the syndromes of congenital adrenal hyperplasia, with emphasis on management of the pediatric patient. 5 refs.

Hamilton W: Congenital adrenal hyperplasia. *Clin Endocrinol Metab,* 1:503–547, 1972.
A detailed review of these syndromes, with practical comments on long-term therapy and surgical correction. 92 refs.

New MI: Congenital adrenal hyperplasia. *Pediatr Clin North Am,* 15:395–407, 1968.
A brief but useful review of these disorders. 26 refs.

Bongiovanni AM and Root AW: The adrenogenital syndrome. *N Engl J Med,* 268:1,283–1,289; 1,342–1,351; 1,391–1,399; 1963.
A classic, complete and still relevant review of the various types of congenital adrenal hyperplasia, written before the days of many plasma steroid measurements. 161 refs.

Lippe BM, LaFranchi SH, Lavin N et al.: Serum 17α-hydroxyprogesterone, progesterone, estradiol and testosterone in the

diagnosis and management of congenital adrenal hyperplasia. ***J Pediatr,*** **85:782–787, 1974.**
The authors evaluated the usefulness of plasma steroid measurements in the control of congenital adrenal hyperplasia with glucocorticoids, compared with traditional assessments. In five new patients, the 17-hydroxyprogesterone and progesterone measurements were useful in assessing the degree of control. 21 refs.

Urban MD, Lee PA and Migeon CJ: Adult height and fertility in men with congenital virilizing adrenal hyperplasia. ***N Engl J Med,*** **299:1,392–1,396, 1978.**
30 men with congenital adrenal hyperplasia treated to varying degrees were evaluated: their mean height was significantly lower than average. Only 2 of 20 patients had abnormal sperm counts; more than 75 percent had fathered children. 29 refs.

Korth-Schutz S, Virdis R, Saenger P et al.: Serum androgens as a continuing index of adequacy of treatment of congenital adrenal hyperplasia. ***J Clin Endocrinol Metab,*** **46:452–458, 1978.**
Control of androgen levels by glucocorticoid treatment was assessed in 19 girls and 17 boys with congenital adrenal hyperplasia. Elevated androstenedione levels correlated with poor control (as assessed by traditional measures) in both sexes. 21 refs.

Klingensmith GJ, Garcia SC, Jones HW Jr. et al.: Glucocorticoid treatment of girls with congenital adrenal hyperplasia: Effects on height, sexual maturation and fertility. ***J Pediatr,*** **90:996–1,004, 1977.**
The authors evaluated 98 females with congenital adrenal hyperplasia of either the 11β- or 21-hydroxylase type. Early treatment promoted attainment of normal adult height. The fertility rate in patients first treated between ages 6 through 20 was 64 percent; all babies required Cesarean delivery. Patient compliance and changing steroid requirements were the major problems with treatment. 33 refs.

Riddick DH and Hammond CB: Long-term steroid therapy in patients with adrenogenital syndrome. ***Obstet Gynecol,*** **45:15–20, 1975.**
26 patients with congenital adrenal hyperplasia diagnosed before age 2 were evaluated. Initial gender assignment was incorrect in six, due to incorrect buccal smears in five. Mean height was below the fiftieth percentile, but otherwise the

patients developed in a near-normal way on steroid therapy. 26 refs.

Pheochromocytoma

Engelman K: Phaeochromocytoma. ***Clin Endocrinol Metab,*** **6:769–797, 1977.**
A complete review of the clinical features, diagnosis, management and therapy of this disorder by a major writer in the field. 45 refs.

Van Way CW III, Scott HW Jr., Page DL and Rhamy RK: Pheochromocytoma. ***Curr Probl Surg,*** **1–59, 1974.**
A detailed review of the surgical approach to patients with either sporadic pheochromocytoma or those associated with MEN 2. 161 refs.

Sjoerdsma A, Engelman K, Waldmann TA et al.: Pheochromocytoma: Current concepts of diagnosis and treatment. ***Ann Intern Med,*** **65:1,302–1,326, 1966.**
An older review of diagnostic criteria, volume status and medical, anesthetic and surgical management of patients with pheochromocytoma. 29 refs.

Gifford RW, Kvale WF, Maher FT et al.: Clinical features, diagnosis and treatment of pheochromocytoma: A review of 76 cases. ***Mayo Clin Proc,*** **39:281–302, 1964.**
This somewhat dated study describes the clinical features of 76 patients with pheochromocytoma at 1 clinic. The most common presenting complaints were headache (25 patients), excessive sweating (18) and attacks or spells (8). 23 refs.

Gitlow SE, Mendlowitz M and Bertani LM: The biochemical techniques for detecting and establishing the presence of a pheochromocytoma: A review of ten years' experience. ***Am J Cardiol,*** **26:270–279, 1970.**
The authors review the diagnostic tests used in 92 patients with proved pheochromocytoma: total metanephrine was always elevated in the patients but also occasionally in the controls; VMA excretion was within normal limits in 3 percent of the patients. Other diagnostic maneuvers are discussed. 70 refs.

Bravo EL, Tarazi RC, Gifford RW and Stewart BH: Circulating and urinary catecholamines in pheochromocytoma. ***N Engl J Med,*** **301:682–686, 1979.**
The authors evaluated diagnostic tests in 24 patients with pheochromocytoma and 40 controls. False-negative plasma

catecholamine values were present in 1 of 23 patients with pheochromocytoma, as opposed to urinary VMA levels in 11 of 22 patients and urinary metanephrines in 5 of 22 patients. 20 refs.

Page LB, Raker JW and Berberich FR: Pheochromocytoma with predominant epinephrine secretion. ***Am J Med*****, 47:648–652, 1969.**
The authors describe a patient with a predominantly epinephrine-secreting pheochromocytoma, and describe the clinical features of 6 other cases: 100 percent had profound hypotension and tachycardia, and perspiration, nausea, vomiting and abdominal pain were present in 86 percent. 14 refs.

Thrall JH: Adrenal scintigraphy. ***Semin Nucl Med*****, 8:23–41, 1978.**
An interesting review of the uses of adrenal scintigraphy with ^{131}I-19-iodocholesterol. Patterns of tracer uptake in various adrenal functional and structural abnormalities are discussed. 52 refs.

Zelch JV, Meaney TF and Belhobek GH: Radiologic approach to the patient with suspected pheochromocytoma. ***Radiology*****, 111:279–284, 1974.**
The authors performed angiography on 34 patients with 37 pheochromocytomas, of which 23 were in the right adrenal, 8 in the left and 6 ectopic. 53 percent of patients became hypertensive during arteriography; severe hypertension was controlled by intravenous phentolamine. 30 percent of tumors were difficult to visualize by arteriography, whereas selective venography was of benefit. 17 refs.

Rossi P, Young IS and Panke WF: Techniques, usefulness and hazards of arteriography of pheochromocytoma: Review of 99 cases. ***JAMA*****, 205:547–553, 1968.**
The authors report 12 cases of pheochromocytoma localized by arteriography and describe 87 more from the literature. Of the 99 cases, mortality was 3 percent; all 3 deaths occurred during translumbar examinations. The authors recommend pretreatment with phenoxybenzamine three to seven days before the procedure. 23 refs.

Ross EJ, Prichard BNC, Kaufman L et al.: Preoperative and operative management of patients with phaeochromocytoma. ***Br Med J*****, 1:191–198, 1967.**
The authors describe their use of adrenergic blockers in 30 operations in 27 patients with pheochromocytoma. They advocate several days of preoperative treatment with phenox-

ybenzamine and propranolol as well as their use intraoperatively. 42 refs.

Remine WH, Chong GC, VanHeerden JA et al.: Current management of pheochromocytoma. ***Ann Surg,*** **179:740–748, 1974.**
The Mayo Clinic series of 138 cases of pheochromocytoma is presented. Of these, 54 percent were women; hypertension was present in 91 percent, but was paroxysmal in only 42 percent. 10 percent of the tumors were ectopic. The authors used both pre- and intraoperative phenoxybenzamine and propranolol with good results; operative mortality was three percent. 13 percent of patients had malignant lesions. 27 refs.

Glenn F and Gray GF: Functional tumors of the organs of Zuckerkandl. ***Ann Surg,*** **183:578–586, 1976.**
The authors describe 4 cases of pheochromocytoma of the organ of Zuckerkandl, and reviewed 46 more cases in the literature. Most patients presented with typical symptoms of pheochromocytoma, although occasionally patients presented with symptoms arising from a retroperitoneal mass. The surgical management of these tumors is discussed. 60 refs.

Hyperaldosteronism

Bravo EL: Regulation of aldosterone secretion: Current concepts and newer aspects. ***Adv Nephrol,*** **7:105–120, 1977.**
A recent review of aldosterone secretory physiology. 64 refs.

Kaplan NN: Adrenal causes of hypertension. ***Arch Intern Med,*** **133:1,001–1,006, 1974.**
The author reviews the adrenal causes of hypertension, including Cushing's syndrome, primary aldosteronism, congenital adrenal hyperplasia and pheochromocytoma. He presents a scheme for evaluation of patients with hypertension and hypokalemia. 49 refs.

Weinberger MH, Grim CE, Hollifield JW et al.: Primary aldosteronism. Diagnosis, localization and treatment. ***Ann Intern Med,*** **90:386–395, 1979.**
A brief but thorough recent review of primary hyperaldosteronism, with special emphasis on newer techniques of tumor localization. The use of these techniques in 51 patients is discussed. 39 refs.

Cain JP, Tuck ML, Williams GH et al.: The regulation of aldosterone secretion in primary aldosteronism. ***Am J Med,*** **53:627–637, 1972.**

The authors describe 20 patients with primary hyperaldosteronism with hypertension, hypokalemia and low renin activity. Aldosterone secretion was affected by ACTH, potassium and angiotensin II, but not by alterations in plasma volume (and thus renin activity). 49 refs.

Ferriss JB, Beevers DG, Brown JJ et al.: Clinical, biochemical and pathological features of low-renin ("primary") hyperaldosteronism. ***Am Heart J*, 95:375–388, 1978.**
In the first of a three-part series on this disorder, the authors review the features of 136 patients: of these, 64 percent were women. Hypokalemia was persistent in 51 percent and intermittent in 38 percent; it was present in all 62 patients with a proved adenoma. Most patients were alkalotic. 117 refs.

Ferriss JB, Beevers DG, Brown JJ et al.: Low renin ("primary") hyperaldosteronism. Differential diagnosis and distinction of subgroups within the syndrome. ***Am Heart J*, 95:641–658, 1978.**
A recent, thorough review of the syndromes of hyperaldosteronism. They emphasize the differential diagnosis of hypertension with hypokalemia, and discuss the advantages of newer diagnostic techniques. 190 refs.

Ferriss JB, Beevers DG, Boddy K et al.: The treatment of low-renin ("primary") hyperaldosteronism. ***Am Heart J*, 96:97–109, 1978.**
The authors discuss the medical and surgical management of this condition. Surgery was performed in 64 patients, 48 of whom had a single adenoma; the results are compared to medical therapy with spironolactone (95 patients), amiloride (18) and dexamethazone (19). 75 refs.

White EA, Schambelan M, Post CR et al.: Use of computed tomography in diagnosing the cause of primary aldosteronism. ***N Engl J Med*, 303:1,503–1,507, 1980.**
Of 22 patients evaluated by computed abdominal tomography for primary aldosteronism, a unilateral mass was seen in 12 patients, and surgically confirmed in 11. Six patients with mild disease had normal or bilaterally enlarged adrenals and were not explored. 37 refs.

Hogan MJ, McRae J, Schambelan M and Biglieri EG: Location of aldosterone-producing adenomas with ^{131}I-19-iodocholesterol. ***N Engl J Med*, 294:410–414, 1976.**
Of 27 patients with hypertension and apparent abnormalities of aldosterone regulation, ^{131}I-19-iodocholesterol imaging revealed asymmetric adrenal uptake in 10. 8 of these patients

had adenomas at operation; the false-positive rate was 1 in 13. 27 refs.

Conn JW, Cohen EL and Herwig KR: The dexamethazone-modified adrenal scintiscan in hyporeninemic aldosteronism (tumor versus hyperplasia). A comparison with adrenal venography and adrenal venous aldosterone. ***J Lab Clin Med*****, 88:841–856, 1976.**
The authors used the dexamethazone-modified adrenal scintiscan to distinguish among 26 patients with hyperaldosteronism. The correct side of the adenoma was predicted in 88 percent of 17 cases; it predicted hyperplasia in 5 of 9 patients explored. It was superior to venography and venous aldosterone measurements in the authors' hands. 19 refs.

Kahn PC, Kelleher D, Egdahl RH and Melby JC: Adrenal arteriography and venography in primary aldosteronism. ***Radiology*****, 101:71–78, 1971.**
The use of adrenal arteriography, venography and venous aldosterone sampling is described in 20 patients with primary hyperaldosteronism. Success rates for correctly diagnosing the lesion were 60 percent, 80 percent and 85 percent, respectively. Adrenal hemorrhage occurred in three patients at venography. 11 refs.

Scoggins BA, Oddie CJ, Hare WSC and Coghlan JP: Preoperative lateralization of aldosterone-producing tumours in primary aldosteronism. ***Ann Intern Med*****, 76:891–897, 1972.**
The authors describe the use of adrenal venous catheterization in the evaluation of primary hyperaldosteronism. Of 11 patients, the diagnosis was made correctly in 10; the final patient had bilateral adenomas. 36 refs.

Beevers DG, Brown JJ, Ferriss JB et al.: The use of spironolactone in the diagnosis and the treatment of hypertension associated with mineralocorticoid excess. ***Am Heart J*****, 86:404–414, 1973.**
The authors briefly review the syndromes of hyperaldosteronism, and describe the appropriate use of spironolactone in each setting. 114 refs.

Hunt TK, Schambelan M and Biglieri EG: Selection of patients and operative approach in primary aldosteronism. ***Ann Surg*****, 182:353–361, 1975.**
The authors review the indications for surgery in primary hyperaldosteronism. In 81 patients with this disorder, surgery resulted in normotension in about 60 percent of 62 patients

with unilateral adenomas. Results were poor in patients with hyperplasia. 13 refs.

Ferriss JB, Brown JJ, Fraser R et al.: Results of adrenal surgery in patients with hypertension, aldosterone excess and low plasma renin concentration. ***Br Med J*, 1:135–138, 1975.**
The authors performed adrenal surgery on 50 patients with primary hyperaldosteronism. Of 38 patients from whom an adenoma was removed, 19 became normotensive; only 2 of 10 with hyperplasia became normotensive. Spironolactone was suggested as long-term treatment for nontumor patients. 23 refs.

Hypoaldosteronism

Phelps KR, Lieberman RL, Oh MS and Carroll HJ: Pathophysiology of the syndrome of hyporeninemic hypoaldosteronism. ***Metabolism*, 29:186–199, 1980.**
A brief, recent review of this poorly understood syndrome. 142 refs.

Schambelan M and Sebastian A: Hyporeninemic hypoaldosteronism. ***Adv Intern Med*, 24:385–405, 1979.**
A recent review of this disorder, based on the authors' review of 22 cases. Most patients had hyperkalemia, hyperchloremic acidosis and depressed creatinine clearance; six patients had diabetes. 62 refs.

Biglieri EG: A perspective on aldosterone abnormalities. ***Clin Endocrinol*, 5:399–410, 1976.**
A brief review of clinical states with high, normal and low aldosterone production. 68 refs.

Michelis MF and Murdaugh HV: Selective hypoaldosteronism. An editorial revisited after 15 years. ***Am J Med*, 59:1–5, 1975.**
A brief review of this problem, with emphasis on the heterogeneity of causes. 27 refs.

Sebastian A, Schambelan M, Lindenfield S and Morris RC Jr.: Amelioration of metabolic acidosis with fludrocortisone therapy in hyporeninemic hypoaldosteronism. ***N Engl J Med*, 297:576–583, 1977.**
The authors treated four patients with renal insufficiency and hypoaldosteronism with fludrocortisone. Both the hyperkalemia and metabolic acidosis were corrected by this means. 38 refs.

DeLeiva A, Christlieb AR, Melby JC et al.: Big renin and biosynthetic defect of aldosterone in diabetes mellitus. *N Engl J Med*, 295:639–643, 1976.
Two patients with isolated hypoaldosteronism and diabetes are described; both had persistent hyperkalemia. In both patients, an enzymatic defect in aldosterone synthesis was noted, in addition to the possible formation of an abnormal, "big" renin by the kidneys. 64 refs.

Glucocorticoid Therapy

Axelrod L: Glucocorticoid therapy. *Medicine*, 55:39–65, 1976.
A complete, recent review of glucocorticoid therapy, with emphasis on evaluation of pituitary-adrenal suppression, steroid withdrawal and alternate day therapy. 188 refs.

Melby JC: Systemic corticosteroid therapy: Pharmacology and endocrinologic considerations. *Ann Intern Med*, 81:505–512, 1974.
The authors reviews the physiologic actions of glucocorticoids, some of their pharmacologic properties, and the effects of dosage schedules on pharmacologic effects and adrenal suppression. 14 refs.

Baxter JD and Forsham PH: Tissue effects of glucocorticoids. *Am J Med*, 53:573–589, 1972.
The effects of glucocorticoids on tissues are reviewed, with emphasis on mechanism and specificity of action, metabolic effects and pharmacologic effects. 172 refs.

Mikely AW and Tyler FH: Potency and duration of action of glucocorticoids. Effects of hydrocortisone, prednisone and dexamethasone on human pituitary–adrenal function. *Am J Med*, 63:200–207, 1977.
The authors investigated biologic potency and plasma half-lives of hydrocortisone, prednisone, and dexamethasone in eight normal subjects, and determined great differences among the three in both indices of potency. 63 refs.

Bynee RL: Withdrawal from glucocorticoid therapy. *N Engl J Med*, 295:330–332, 1976.
A brief discussion of this common clinical problem. The author presents a practical protocol for steroid withdrawal using the response to the short ACTH test as a guide. 24 refs.

Ammatruda TT Jr, Hurst MM and Hopo DS: Certain endocrine and metabolic facets of the steroid withdrawal syndrome. *J Clin Endocrinol Metab*, 25:1207–1217, 1965.

The steroid withdrawal syndrome is described in 22 patients from whom exogenous steroids were removed. They developed anorexia, nausea, lethargy, arthralgia, weakness, desquamation and weight loss. In 13 patients, baseline plasma and serum steroids and response to ACTH were the same as in control subjects. 38 refs.

Graber AL, Ney RL, Nicholson WE et al.: Natural history of pituitary-adrenal recovery following long-term suppression with corticosteroids. ***J Clin Endocrinol Metab*, 25:11–16, 1965.**
The authors describe the time course of recovery of the glucocorticoid axis following exogenous steroid treatment in 14 patients. The pituitary recovered first, but cortisol secretion became normal only after several months of high ACTH levels. 20 refs.

Livanou T, Ferriman D and James VHT: Recovery of hypothalamo-pituitary-adrenal function after corticosteroid therapy. ***Lancet*, 2:856–859, 1967.**
The authors studied the response of plasma 11-hydroxycorticosteroid levels to insulin-induced hypoglycemia in 21 normal subjects and 72 patients either on steroids or after stopping steroids for varying lengths of time. The response did not become normal for 1 year in some cases. 13 refs.

Walton J, Watson BS and Ney RL: Alternate day versus shorter interval steroid administration. ***Arch Intern Med*, 126:601–607, 1970.**
When identical doses of steroids were given every 8 hours instead of every other day to 9 normal volunteers, urinary excretion of nitrogen was greater in the former group. The hyperglycemic effect of the alternate day dosage disappeared before each successive dose. 20 refs.

Ackerman GL and Nolan CM: Adrenocortical responsiveness after alternate-day corticosteroid therapy. ***N Engl J Med*, 278:405–409, 1968.**
The responsiveness of plasma 17-hydroxycorticosteroid levels to insulin-induced hypogylcemia was assessed in 10 patients on long-term, alternate day prednisone therapy. The response was similar to that in a control group, and superior to a group of patients on daily steroids. 14 refs.

Bongiovanni AM and McPadden AJ: Steroids during pregnancy and possible fetal consequences. ***Fertil Steril*, 11:181–186, 1960.**
A short review of the harmful effects of steroids taken during pregnancy. 40 refs.

GONADAL DISORDERS (EXCLUDING INFERTILITY AND NONSECRETING TUMORS OF REPRODUCTIVE ORGANS)

Physiology and Diagnosis

Shaw RW: Neuroendocrinology of the menstrual cycle in humans. ***Clin Endocrinol Metab*****, 7:531–559, 1979.**
A recent, thorough review of this topic, with emphasis on the various feedback loops operating during the cycle, and recent advances in the physiology and pharmacology of GNRH. About 130 refs.

Boyar RM: Control of the onset of puberty. ***Annu Rev Med*****, 29:509–520, 1978.**
A very interesting review of the hormonal events producing puberty, and some of their disorders. 37 refs.

Forest MG, DePeretti E and Bertrand J: Hypothalamic-pituitary-gonadal relationships in man from birth to puberty. ***Clin Endocrinol*****, 5:551–569, 1976.**
A brief review of gonadotropin physiology in neonatal life and childhood with comments on the changes that occur as puberty approaches. About 126 refs.

Yen SSC, Lasley BL, Wang CF et al.: The operating characteristics of the hypothalamic-pituitary system during the menstrual cycle and observations of biological action of somatostatin. ***Recent Prog Horm Res*****, 31:321–363, 1975.**
A long and complex review of the authors' studies on the neuroendocrinology of the menstrual cycle. About 120 refs.

Shaw RW: Tests of the hypothalamic-pituitary-ovarian axis. ***Clin Obstet Gynecol*****, 3:485–503, 1976.**
The author reviews the practical assessment of this axis, including gonadotropin and steroid measurements, the LHRH test and tests of hypothalamic function based on normal feedback controls. 79 refs.

Faiman C, Winter JSD and Reyes FI: Patterns of gonadotropins and gonadal steroids throughout life. ***Clin Obstet Gynecol*****, 3:467–483, 1976.**
This brief review does just what the title says, with descriptions of these hormones during fetal life, infancy, adolescence, the reproductive years and the menopausal years. 57 refs.

Chan L and O'Malley BW: Mechanism of action of the sex-

steroid hormones. ***N Engl J Med*****, 294:1,322–1,328; 1,372–1,381; 1,430–1,437; 1976.**
An extensive review which incorporates many of the recent advances in this field. 301 refs.

Franchimont P, Valcke JC and Lambotte R: Female gonadal dysfunction. ***Clin Endocrinol Metab*****, 3:533–556, 1974.**
An overview of disorders of female reproductive endocrinology, with an emphasis on practical diagnosis of common disorders. 43 refs.

Coutts JRT: Hormone production by the ovary. ***Clin Obstet Gynecol*****, 3:63–87, 1976.**
A recent review of ovarian endocrinology, focusing on the ovary during reproductive life. 81 refs.

Jeffcoate SL: The control of testicular function in the adult. ***Clin Endocrinol Metab*****, 4:521–543, 1975.**
The author reviews hypothalamic-pituitary-testicular endocrine relationships. 97 refs.

Secondary Amenorrhea (General) (See Also Galactorrhea-Amenorrhea Syndromes, Anorexia Nervosa and Hypopituitarism)

Nakano R, Hashiba N, Kotsuji F and Tojo S: A schematic approach to the work-up of amenorrhea. ***Fertil Steril*****, 28:229–236, 1977.**
The authors evaluated 33 amenorrheic patients and 7 controls by means of a progestin-withdrawal test, a cyclic estrogen and progestin test, an LHRH test and a gonadotropin loading test, and came up with a scheme for evaluating amenorrhea on the basis of these results. 22 refs.

Kletzky OA, Davajan V, Nakamura RM and Mishell DR Jr.: Classification of secondary amenorrhea based on distinct hormonal patterns. ***J Clin Endocrinol Metab*****, 41:660–668, 1975.**
Gonadotropin pulsations were measured in 21 patients with secondary amenorrhea, and allowed the authors to distinguish among polycystic ovary syndrome, hypothalamic-pituitary dysfunction or failure and ovarian failure. 26 refs.

Farber M: Evaluation of secondary amenorrhea. ***Clin Obstet Gynecol*****, 20:805–813, 1977.**
A short review in which a scheme for evaluating secondary amenorrhea is presented. 31 refs.

Kletzky OA, Davajan V, Nakamura RM et al.: Clinical categorization of patients with secondary amenorrhea using pro-

gesterone-induced uterine bleeding and measurement of serum gonadotropin levels. ***Am J Obstet Gynecol*, 121:695–703, 1975.**
Of 90 women with secondary amenorrhea, 63 had withdrawal bleeding in response to progesterone; of these, patients with high LH (21) were thought to have polycystic ovary syndrome, the remainder (42) having hypothalamic-pituitary dysfunction. In the remaining patients, 12 had elevated FSH, indicating primary ovarian failure, and 15 patients had hypothalamic dysfunction. 24 refs.

Rebar RW, Erickson GF and Yen SSC: Idiopathic premature ovarian failure: Clinical and endocrine characteristics. ***Fertil Steril*, 37:35–41, 1982.**
Of 26 patients with presumed early ovarian failure, based on elevated gonadotropin levels and other findings, several later showed evidence of ovulation and one became pregnant. The authors stress that ovulation is possible in some patients falsely diagnosed as having permanent premature ovarian failure. 24 refs.

Lachelin GCL and Yen SSC: Hypothalamic chronic anovulation. ***Am J Obstet Gynecol*, 130:825–831, 1978.**
11 patients with amenorrhea, psychological problems and normal gonadotropins were evaluated. Few and minor hormonal changes were noted, and periods often returned after psychological counseling. 26 refs.

Klein SM and Garcia CR: Asherman's syndrome: A critique and current review. ***Fertil Steril*, 24:722–735, 1973.**
An extensive review of this relatively uncommon cause of secondary amenorrhea. 33 refs.

Hirsutism and Virilism (General)

Givens JR: Hirsutism and hyperandrogenism. ***Adv. Intern Med*, 21:221–247, 1976.**
An extremely readable review of this topic, including discussions of androgen physiology in women, androgen levels in hirsute women, the concepts of ovarian and adrenal hyperandrogenism and the diagnostic work-up of hirsute patients. 100 refs.

Farber M, Millan VG, Tukson RN and Mitchell GW Jr.: Diagnostic evaluation of hirsutism in women. ***Clin Obstet Gynecol*, 20:1–9, 1977.**
A brief, readable review of recent advances in the diagnostic evaluation of hirsutism. The authors maintain that selective

adrenal and ovarian venous catheterization should be part of the evaluation of many patients with hirsutism. 33 refs.

Genazzani AR, Pecciarini-Snickars L, Franchi F et al.: Diagnostic approach to the hirsute patient. ***Horm Res*, 9:379–393, 1978.**
A brief, recent review of androgen production and metabolism in women, and the diagnostic approach to the hirsute patient. 42 refs.

Kirschner MA, Zucker IR and Jesperson D: Idiopathic hirsutism—An ovarian abnormality. ***N Engl J Med*, 294:637–640, 1976.**
44 women with unexplained hirsutism were evaluated. All had increased testosterone production rates; 42 patients had increased ovarian vein androgens, including 20 patients whose serum androgens were suppressed by dexamethazone administration. 26 refs.

Lipsett M, Wessler S and Avioli LV: The differential diagnosis of hirsutism and virilism. ***Arch Intern Med*, 132:616–619, 1973.**
A brief review of the steps to be taken by the internist in the evaluation of patients with hirsutism or virilism. 14 refs.

The Polycystic Ovary Syndrome

Yen SSC: The polycystic ovary syndrome. ***Clin Endocrinol*, 12:177–208, 1980.**
An excellent recent review of this disorder by a prominent researcher in the field. Recent information about the syndrome's pathophysiology is discussed in detail; little is said about treatment. 131 refs.

Goldzieher JW and Axelrod LR: Clinical and biochemical features of polycystic ovarian disease. ***Fertil Steril*, 14:631–653, 1963.**
A detailed but now somewhat out of date review of this syndrome, with data tabulated from 187 references and 1,079 cases. The results of wedge resection are discussed, and include a 63 percent incidence of pregnancy! 97 refs.

Rebar R, Judd HL, Yen SSC et al.: Characterization of the inappropriate gonadotropin secretion in polycystic ovary syndrome. ***J Clin Invest*, 57:1,320–1,329, 1976.**
In 24 patients with biopsy proven PCO, LH levels tended to be high, and FSH levels tended to be low and not pulsatile. LH release after LRF was exaggerated, and LH and FSH responses to clomiphene were normal. The authors postulate a primary ovarian defect. 45 refs.

DeVane GW, Czekala NM, Judd HL and Yen SSC: Circulating gonadotropins, estrogens and androgens in polycystic ovarian disease. ***Am J Obstet Gynecol*****, 121:496–500, 1965.**
Plasma hormone levels at day 2 through 4 of the menstrual cycle were compared in 19 women with laparoscopically-documented polycystic ovary disease (PCO) and 10 normal women. Plasma testosterone, LH, androstenedione, estrone and dehidroepiandrosterone sulfate were all significantly elevated in patients with PCO. 26 refs.

Judd HL, Rigg LA, Anderson DC and Yen SSC: The effects of ovarian wedge resection on circulating gonadotropin and ovarian steroid levels in patients with polycystic ovary syndrome. ***J Clin Endocrinol Metab*****, 43:347–355, 1976.**
Eight patients undergoing wedge resection for PCO were studied. The operation caused a temporary decrease in androstenedione production and a sustained decrease in testosterone production, but did not directly affect gonadotropin levels. 42 refs.

Yen SSC, Vela P and Ryan KJ: Effect of clomiphene citrate in polycystic ovary syndrome: Relationship between serum gonadotropin and corpus luteum formation. ***J Clin Endocrinol Metab*****, 31:7–13, 1970.**
7 patients with PCO were treated with clomiphene for 8 cycles, resulting in most cases in an increase in gonadotropin levels, followed by an LH surge about 12 days after beginning treatment. Seven of eight cycles were ovulatory. 25 refs.

Raj SG, Berger MJ, Grimes EM and Taymor ML: The use of gonadotropins for the induction of ovulation in women with polycystic ovarian disease. ***Fertil Steril*****, 28:1,280–1,284, 1977.**
10 patients with PCO and infertility were treated with either pure human FSH or mixed postmenopausal human gonadotropin. FSH administration resulted in more ovulatory cycles and less hyperstimulation than did FSH and LH administration. 13 refs.

Jafari K, Javaheri G and Ruiz G: Endometrial adenocarcinoma and the Stein-Leventhal syndrome. ***Obstet Gynecol*****, 51:97–100, 1978.**
Six patients with PCO who later developed endometrial carcinoma are described; the authors review 53 other cases from the literature. The patients had a mean age of 28, and the tumors were well-differentiated adenocarcinomas. 21 refs.

Abraham GE and Buster JE: Peripheral and ovarian steroids in ovarian hyperthecosis. ***Obstet Gynecol*****, 47:581–586, 1976.**

Steroids in peripheral and ovarian venous blood were measured in two patients with virilization and ovarian hyperthecosis. Of measured androgens, only testosterone and dihydrotestosterone were elevated, and decreased following oophorectomy. 14 refs.

Judd HL, Scully RE, Herbst AL et al.: Familial hyperthecosis: Comparison of endocrinologic and histologic findings with polycystic ovarian disease. ***Am J Obstet Gynecol,*** **117:976–982, 1973.**
Two sisters with ovarian hyperthecosis had normal LH and low to normal FSH levels, and high levels of testosterone and androstenedione; concentrations of these androgens increased to preoperative levels three months after wedge resection. 33 refs.

Virilizing Tumors of the Ovary

Shane JM and Naftolin F: Aberrant hormone activity by tumors of gynecologic importance. ***Am J Obstet Gynecol,*** **121:133–147, 1975.**
A complete review of hormonal syndromes resulting from gynecologic tumors. 226 refs.

Novak ER and Long JH: Arrhenoblastoma of the ovary. A review of the ovarian tumor registry. ***Am J Obstet Gynecol,*** **92:1,082–1,093, 1965.**
Of 111 cases of arrhenoblastoma reviewed by the authors, 98 had associated virilism and 13 without androgenic effect. Five patients had bilateral tumors; malignant spread could only be diagnosed clinically. 18 refs.

Pedowitz P and O'Brien FB: Arrhenoblastoma of the ovary. Review of the literature and report of two cases. ***Obstet Gynecol,*** **16:62–77, 1960.**
Of 240 cases of arrhenoblastoma collected in this series, 96 percent were unilateral, 16 percent were less than 6 cm in diameter and 21 percent were malignant; 70 percent of patients had amenorrhea, 79 percent had hirsutism and less than half of patients tested had elevated urinary 17-ketosteroids. 193 refs.

Lawson TL and Albarelli JN: Diagnosis of gynecologic pelvic masses by gray scale ultrasonography: Analysis of specificity and accuracy. ***Am J Roentgenol,*** **128:1,003–1,006, 1977.**
Of 251 cases with proven pelvic mass, the authors claim 91 percent accuracy in determining the existence, size, location

and consistency of the mass. Lesions less than two cm in diameter were poorly visualized. 4 refs.

Turner's Syndrome

McDonough P and Byrd JR: Gonadal dysgenesis. ***Clin Obstet Gynecol,*** **20:565–579, 1977.**
A short review of this condition, emphasizing the genetic heterogeneity despite common clinical features, the diagnosis of the syndrome and therapy. 24 refs.

Engel E and Forbes AP: Cytogenetic and clinical findings in 48 patients with congenitally defective or absent ovaries. ***Medicine,*** **44:135–164, 1965.**
The records of 48 patients with congenitally defective or absent ovaries were reviewed; 7 types of cytogenetic abnormalities were noted, including only 16 patients with the classical sex chromosomal complement. Most patients had the clinical features of Turner's syndrome. 89 refs.

Teter J and Boczkowski K: Occurrence of tumors in dysgenetic gonads. ***Cancer,*** **20:1,301–1,310, 1967.**
In 51 patients with gonadal dysgenesis undergoing laparotomy, 10 ovarian tumors were found. 2 occurred in 25 patients with Turner's syndrome, and 8 occurred in 26 cases of gonadal dysgenesis without somatic malformations. Sex chromatin pattern was negative in all 10 patients with tumors. 36 refs.

Samaan NA, Stepanas AV, Danziger J and Trujillo J: Reactive pituitary abnormalities in patients with Klinefelter's and Turner's syndromes. ***Arch Intern Med,*** **139:198–201, 1979.**
Of 10 patients with gonadal dysgenesis, 4 developed enlarged sellas; the other 6 demonstrated abnormal sellar contours on tomography. All had abnormally high FSH levels and response to stimulation; reactive pituitary hyperplasia or adenoma formation is suggested. 27 refs.

Androgen Resistant Syndromes

Griffin JE and Wilson JD: The syndromes of androgen resistance. ***N Engl J Med,*** **302:198–209, 1980.**
An excellent, readable, recent review of these disorders, including newer advances in androgen action, and the clinical disorders of 5α-reductase deficiency, androgen receptor disorders and the syndromes of "receptor-positive androgen resistance". 110 refs.

Aiman J, Griffin JE, Gazak JM et al.: Androgen insensitivity as a cause of infertility in otherwise normal men. ***N Engl J Med*****, 300:223–227, 1979.**
Three men with long standing infertility were found to have elevated plasma testosterone concentrations and decreased binding of dihydrotestosterone to genital-skin fibroblasts, indicating androgen insensitivity as a cause of their infertility. 34 refs.

Griffin JE and Wilson JD: Hereditary male pseudohermaphroditism. ***Clin Obstet Gynecol*****, 5:457–479, 1978.**
A complete recent review of these syndromes, with an emphasis on defects of testosterone synthesis. 53 refs.

Crawford JD, Adams RD, Kliman B et al.: Syndromes of testicular feminization. ***Clin Pediatr*****, 9:165–178, 1970.**
An informal discussion of the diagnosis and management of this syndrome (complete and incomplete) in childhood and adolescence. 32 refs.

Amrhein JA, Klingensmith GJ, Walsh PC et al.: Partial androgen insensitivity. The Reifenstein syndrome revisited. ***N Engl J Med*****, 297:350–356, 1977.**
In eight patients with this syndrome, all had elevated LH and testosterone levels, and normal 5α-reductase activity. Four of five patients had normal cytoplasmic dihydrotestosterone binding, indicating a "post-receptor" defect. 40 refs.

Bowen P, Lee CSN, Migeon CJ et al.: Hereditary male pseudohermaphroditism with hypogonadism, hypospadias and gynecomastia (Reifenstein's syndrome). ***Ann Intern Med*****, 62:252–270, 1965.**
Members of three families with this syndrome are described, having: hypospadias, testicular atrophy with elevated gonadotropin levels, azoospermia, weak virilization and gynecomastia. 31 refs.

Male Hypogonadal Hypogonadism (See Also Hypopituitarism)

Baker HWG and Hudson B: Male gonadal dysfunction. ***Clin Endocrinol Metab*****, 3:507–531, 1974.**
A practical guide to the evaluation and diagnosis of male reproductive disorders, with a major section on male infertility. 36 refs.

Wu FCW, Edmond P, Raab G and Hunter WM: Endocrine

assessment of the subfertile male. ***Clin Endocrinol*, 14:493–507, 1981.**
The authors evaluated 102 patients with low sperm densities (less than 40 × 10^6/ml), and concluded that: The LHRH test is not indicated in the routine evaluation of male subfertility; and testicular biopsy is only indicated when very low sperm counts and normal FSH are present. 41 refs.

Federman DD: Testicular deficiency. ***Adv Intern Med*, 16:81–102, 1970.**
A short but fairly complete review of hypogonadism, with emphasis on pubertal gonadal disturbances. 89 refs.

Paulsen CA, Gordon DL, Carpenter RW et al.: Klinefelter's syndrome and its variants: A hormonal and chromosomal study. ***Recent Prog Horm Res*, 24:321–363, 1968.**
An extensive review of these hypogonadal syndromes, including clinical features, chromosomal studies, biochemical findings and results of testicular biopsy. 261 refs.

Wang C, Baker HWG, Burger HG et al.: Hormonal studies in Klinefelter's syndrome. ***Clin Endocrinol*, 4:399–411, 1975.**
19 patients with Klinefelter's syndrome had low testosterone levels and production, and elevated plasma estradiol, FSH and LH levels. The gonadotropin levels were suppressed by chronic testosterone administration. 41 refs.

Meinhard E, McRae CU and Chisholm GD: Testicular biopsy in evaluation of male infertility. ***Br Med J*, 3:577–581, 1973.**
100 infertile men underwent testicular biopsy; 43 percent had severe tubular lesions, and mild or moderately severe lesions were seen in the remainder. The authors discuss the role of this technique in the evaluation of male hypogonadism and infertility. 11 refs.

Jeffcoate WJ, Lawrence BM, Edwards CRW and Besser GM: Endocrine function in the Prader-Willi syndrome. ***Clin Endocrinol*, 12:81–89, 1980.**
Eight patients with the Prader-Willi syndrome were found to have subnormal responses after LHRH administration, as well as subnormal gonadal responses to HCG. 14 refs.

Feminizing Tumors in Men

Anderson T, Waldmann TA, Javadpour N and Glatstein E: Testicular germ cell neoplasms: Recent advances in diagnosis and therapy. ***Ann Intern Med*, 90:373–385, 1979.**

A recent review of these tumors at the NIH, focusing on markers of germ cell neoplasms, and the immunocytochemistry, staging, surgery, radiation therapy and chemotherapy of testicular tumors. 82 refs.

Peckham MJ and McElwain TJ: Testicular tumours. *Clin Endocrinol Metab*, 4:665–692, 1975.
An extensive review of testicular tumors of all types, with comments on hormone-secreting tumors and treatment. About 86 refs.

Keough B, Hreshchyshyn MM, Moore RH et al.: Urinary gonadotropins in management and prognosis of testicular tumor. *Urology*, 5:496–503, 1975.
The authors assessed the value of HCG measurements in the evaluation of 93 patients with germinal testicular tumors. High urinary HCG levels were associated with nonseminomatous tumors, and a poor prognosis when observed postoperatively. 16 refs.

Gabrilove JL, Sharma DC, Wotiz HH and Dorfman RI: Feminizing adrenocortical tumors in the male: A review of 52 cases including a case report. *Medicine*, 44:37–79, 1965.
The authors review 52 cases of feminizing adrenal tumors in men. Common symptoms and signs were gynecomastia (98 percent), palpable tumor (58 percent), testicular atrophy (52 percent) and diminished libido (48 percent). Most were carcinomas. 106 refs.

Sex Steroid Replacement Therapy

Estrogens (See Also Osteoporosis)

Hilliard GD and Norris HJ: Pathologic effects of oral contraceptives. *Recent Results Cancer Res*, 66:49–71, 1979.
A detailed and recent review of the effects of long-term oral contraceptive use on the tissues of the uterus, fallopian tubes, ovary, vagina and breast, as well as on the development of thromboembolic disease, hypertension and impaired carbohydrate tolerance. 133 refs.

Thomas DB: Role of exogenous female hormones in altering the risk of benign and malignant neoplasms in humans. *Cancer Res*, 38:3,991–4,000, 1978.
A concise review of possible estrogen associated tumors, including cancer of the vagina, endometrium, ovary, cervix, breast and liver. 98 refs.

Mishell DR Jr.: Current status of oral contraceptive steroids. ***Clin Obstet Gynecol*, 19:743–764, 1976.**
An interesting review of oral contraceptive pharmacology, physiology and metabolic effects, with comments on the choice of formulation. 45 refs.

Vana J, Murphy GP, Aronoff BL and Baker HW: Primary liver tumors and oral contraceptives. Results of a survey. ***JAMA*, 238:2,154–2,158, 1977.**
An interesting survey of 378 female and 165 male patients with primary liver tumors. In the men, 92 percent of tumors were malignant, compared to only 44 percent in the women. A history of oral contraceptive use was obtained in 74 percent of women with hepatic cell adenomas. 20 refs.

Weinstein MC: Estrogen use in postmenopausal women—costs, risks and benefits. ***N Engl J Med*, 303:308–316, 1980.**
A cost-benefit analysis of estrogen use in postmenopausal women in which the author concludes that treatment is relatively cost-effective in women with osteoporosis or prior hysterectomy. 39 refs.

Quigley MM and Hammond CB: Estrogen-replacement therapy—Help or hazard? ***N Engl J Med*, 301:646–648, 1979.**
A recent, brief and sensible summary of current indications and contraindications for estrogen replacement therapy. 20 refs.

Ryan KJ, Barrett-Connor E, Federman DD et al.: Estrogen use and postmenopausal women: A National Institutes of Health consensus development conference. ***Ann Intern Med*, 91:921–922, 1979.**
At a meeting of experts in the field, the consensus was that: estrogens decrease menopausal vasomotor symptoms, retard bone loss and do not increase the risk of heart disease, stroke or thromboembolic disease; estrogens also appear to increase the incidence of endometrial, but not breast cancer. No refs.

Weiss NS and Sayvetz TA: Incidence of endometrial cancer in relation to the use of oral contraceptives. ***N Engl J Med*, 302:551–554, 1980.**
The incidence of oral contraceptive use among 117 patients with endometrial cancer was compared to that of 395 controls. The risk was 7.3 times higher than control with one sequential contraceptive; women taking combined pills had a lower cancer risk than controls. 9 refs.

Ishak KG: Hepatic neoplasms associated with contraceptive and anabolic steroids. ***Recent Results Cancer Res*, 66:73–128, 1979.**
A very long, detailed and careful review of hepatic tumors occurring with oral contraceptive use (hepatocellular adenoma and carcinoma) and those occurring with androgen use (hepatocellular carcinoma, rarely adenoma and peliosis hepatitis). 155 refs.

Utian WH: Current status of menopause and postmenopausal estrogen therapy. ***Obstet Gynecol Surv*, 32:193–204, 1977.**
A brief review of the physiology and symptoms of menopause, and the benefits and hazards of estrogen replacement in postmenopausal women. 91 refs.

Hammond CB, Jelovsek FR, Lee KL et al.: Effects of long-term estrogen replacement therapy. I. Metabolic effects. ***Am J Obstet Gynecol*, 133:525–536, 1979.**
The authors reviewed the records of 301 patients treated with replacement estrogen, and 309 untreated patients. Lower rates of cardiovascular disease, hypertension, osteoporosis and fractures were found in the estrogen treated women, while cancer of the endometrium was more common. 31 refs.

Hammond CB, Jelovsek FR, Lee KL et al.: Effects of long-term estrogen replacement therapy. II. Neoplasia. ***Am J Obstet Gynceol*, 133:537–547, 1979.**
In the same group of patients reported in Part I, the risk of developing endometrial carcinoma was increased in the estrogen treated group (but no other cancers). Adding a progestin to the regimen decreased the risk of endometrial cancer. 20 refs.

Androgens

Wilson JD and Griffin JE: The use and misuse of androgens. ***Metabolism*, 29:1,278–1,295, 1980.**
A complete, recent and much needed review of this topic. The authors discuss the pharmacology of available androgens, their use in replacement therapy, their abuse in athletes and their side effects. 224 refs.

Fukutani K, Isurugi K, Takayasu H et al.: Effects of depot testosterone therapy on serum levels of luteinizing hormone and follicle stimulating hormone in patients with Klinefelter's syndrome and hypogonadotropic eunuchoidism. ***J Clin Endocrinol Metab*, 39:856–864, 1974.**
21 patients with Klinefelter's syndrome were studied. The authors found that more frequent testosterone injections were

necessary to suppress gonadotropins in these patients than in normal men. 26 refs.

Bagheri SA and Boyer JL: Peliosis hepatis associated with androgenic-anabolic steroid therapy. A severe form of hepatic injury. ***Ann Intern Med*****, 81:610–618, 1974.**
7 patients on androgens for 2 to 27 months developed peliosis hepatis, generally with hepatomegaly and abnormal liver function. Life-threatening shock or hepatic failure developed in five patients. 22 refs.

Nadell J and Kosek J: Peliosis hepatis. 12 cases associated with oral androgen therapy. ***Arch Pathol Lab Med*****, 101:405–410, 1977.**
12 patients on oxymetholone or fluoxymesterone therapy developed peliosis hepatis. Three patients died of hepatic failure while being treated; in one patient in whom the diagnosis was established by biopsy, the lesion regressed after androgens were stopped. A total of 42 cases from the literature were reviewed. 30 refs.

Ishak KG: Hepatic neoplasms associated with contraceptive and anabolic steroids. ***Recent Results Cancer Res*****, 66:73–128, 1979.**
A very long, detailed and careful review of hepatic tumors occurring with oral contraceptive use (hepatocellular adenoma and carcinoma) and those occurring with androgen use (hepatocellular carcinoma, rarely adenoma and peliosis hepatis). 155 refs.

PARATHYROID DISORDERS AND METABOLIC BONE DISEASE

Physiology and Diagnosis

Harris WH and Heaney RP: Skeletal renewal and metabolic bone disease. ***N Engl J Med*****, 280:193–202; 253–259; 303–311; 1969.**
An extensive review of bone metabolism, metabolic and hormonal effectors of bone resorbtion, and metabolic bone diseases. 128 refs.

Rasmussen H, Bordier P, Kurokawa K et al.: Hormonal control of skeletal and mineral homeostasis. ***Am J Med*****, 56:751–758, 1974.**
A concise review of the effects of PTH, calcitonin and vitamin D metabolites on bone cells. 30 refs.

Lutwak L, Singer FR and Urist MR: ***Ann Intern Med*****, 80:630–644, 1974.**

A UCLA conference in which the discussion included properties of bone structure, the effects of calcitonin and the role of dietary calcium on the skeleton. 96 refs.

Rasmussen H: Ionic and hormonal control of calcium homeostasis. *Am J Med*, 50:567–588, 1971.
An extensive review of calcium homeostasis with emphasis on hormonal effects on bone cells. 164 refs.

Raisz LG: Physiologic and pharmacologic regulation of bone resorption. *N Engl J Med*, 282:909–916, 1970.
A brief review of physiologic and pharmacologic control of bone remodelling, now somewhat dated. 59 refs.

Parfitt AM: The actions of parathyroid hormone on bone: Relation to bone remodeling and turnover, calcium homeostasis and metabolic bone disease (Parts I-IV). *Metabolism*, 25:809–844; 909–955; 1,033–1,069; 1,157–1,188; 1976.
An amazingly complete review of the skeletal effects of parathyroid hormone, with comments on diagnosis and clinical features of most types of metabolic bone disease. 171 refs.; 303 refs.; 211 refs.; 209 refs.

Diaz-Buxo JA and Knox FG: Effects of parathyroid hormone on renal function. *Mayo Clin Proc*, 50:537–541, 1975.
A brief review of PTH effects on renal handling of calcium, phosphate, amino acids and in acid-base disturbances. 96 refs.

Robinson CJ: The physiology of parathyroid hormone. *Clin Endocrinol Metab*, 3:389–417, 1974.
A concise review of the effects of PTH on kidney, gut and bone, with emphasis on normal physiology. 187 refs.

Parsons JA and Potts JT Jr.: Physiology and chemistry of parathyroid hormone. *Clin Endocrinol Metab*, 1:33–78, 1972.
An extensive review of the action of parathyroid hormone on bone, small intestine and other actions, with comments on its chemistry and radioimmunoassay. About 198 refs.

Jowsey J: Quantitative microradiography: A new approach in the evaluation of metabolic bone disease. *Am J Med*, 40:485–491, 1966.
A brief editorial describing quantitative analysis of bone biopsy specimens in the diagnosis and management of metabolic bone disease. 23 refs.

Holick MF and Clark MB: The photobiogenesis and metabolism of vitamin D. *Fed Proc*, 37:2,567–2,574, 1978.

A brief review of vitamin D chemistry, with emphasis on its generation from precursors in skin. 94 refs.

DeLuca HF: Vitamin D metabolism and function. ***Arch Intern Med,*** **138:836–847, 1978.**
A complete, current review of what is known about vitamin D metabolism and relevant clinical states by one of the foremost researchers in the field. 121 refs.

Haussler MR and McCain TA: Basic and clinical concepts related to vitamin D metabolism and action. ***N Engl J Med,*** **297:974–983; 1,041–1,050, 1977.**
A complete and up-to-date review of vitamin D action, with emphasis in the second part on assays of vitamin D metabolites and the therapy of relevant clinical disorders. 203 refs.

Hyperparathyroidism (See Also Hypercalcemia and Parathyroid Carcinoma)

General

Heath H III, Hodgson SF and Kennedy MA: Primary hyperparathyroidism. Incidence, morbidity and potential economic impact in a community. ***N Engl J Med,*** **302:189–193, 1980.**
The annual incidence of new cases of primary hyperparathyroidism in Rochester, Minn. rose from 7.8 per 100,000 (1965 to 1974) to 51.1 per 100,000 (after 1974). The proportion of patients without symptoms rose dramatically. The authors discuss the implications of these findings. (See accompanying editorial.) 37 refs.

Watson L: Primary hyperparathyroidism. ***Clin Endocrinol Metab,*** **3:215–235, 1974.**
A concise review of most aspects of this disorder. 39 refs.

Mallette LE, Bilezikian JP, Heath DA et al.: Primary hyperparathyroidism: Clinical and biochemical features. ***Medicine,*** **53:127–146, 1974.**
The authors review 57 cases of primary hyperparathyroidism. The most common features were hypertension, weakness, fatigability, renal colic, mental disturbances, constipation and epigastric pain. Eight patients had osteitis fibrosa cystica. 70 refs.

Aurbach GD, Mallette LE, Patten BM et al.: Hyperparathyroidism: Recent studies. ***Ann Intern Med,*** **79:566–581, 1973.**
A NIH conference on primary hyperparathyroidism, in which

the authors discuss the general clinical features of 57 cases, the neurologic findings of 16 cases and the angiographic localization of parathyroid adenomas. 48 refs.

Genant HK, Heck LL, Lanzl LH et al.: Primary hyperparathyroidism: A comprehensive study of clinical, biochemical and radiographic manifestations. ***Radiology*****, 109:513–524, 1973.**
Of 65 patients with primary hyperparathyroidism, 10 percent had phalangeal subperiosteal reabsorbtion with conventional x-rays; on fine-detail radiography, most patients had some subperiosteal reabsorbtion, and most had osteopenia as determined by bone mineral density. 69 refs.

Purnell DC, Smith LH, Scholz DA et al.: Primary hyperparathyroidism: A prospective clinical study. ***Am J Med,*** **50:670–678, 1971.**
Of 322 patients with probable hyperparathyroidism, 171 of 191 patients with indications for surgery had confirmed primary hyperparathyroidism at surgery. Of 147 patients not undergoing surgery, 21 developed one of the indications for operation in the 30 month follow-up period. 15 refs.

Christensson T, Hellström K and Wengle B: Hypercalcemia and primary hyperparathyroidism. Prevalence in patients receiving thiazaides as detected in a health screen. ***Arch Intern Med,*** **137:1,138–1,142, 1977.**
Of 95 patients with asymptomatic hypercalcemia picked up during a screen of 15,903 persons, 20 were taking thiazides. Of these 20, 14 were found to have parathyroid adenomas at neck exploration; 5 patients became normocalcemic after thiazides were stopped. 19 refs.

Marx SJ, Spiegel AM, Brown EM et al.: Divalent cation metabolism. Familial hypocalcemic hypercalcemia versus typical primary hyperparathyroidism. ***Am J Med,*** **65:235–242, 1978.**
23 patients with familial idiopathic hypocalciuric hypercalcemia demonstrated higher serum magnesium and lower renal calcium and magnesium excretions than 63 patients with primary hyperparathyroidism. Plasma proteins, and ionized and bound calcium fractions were similar in the two group. 28 refs.

Cogan MG, Covey CM, Arieff AI et al.: Central nervous system manifestations of hyperparathyroidism. ***Am J Med,*** **65:963–970, 1978.**
13 patients with hyperparathyroidism were compared neurologically with 6 undergoing neck surgery for other reasons. The hyperparathyroid patients had abnormal EEGs, and those

with secondary hyperparathyroidism had abnormal levels of intellectual function; both were corrected by surgery. 26 refs.

Martin KJ, Hruska KA, Freitag JJ et al.: The peripheral metabolism of parathyroid hormone. ***N Engl J Med*****, 301:1,092–1,098, 1979.**
A brief and up-to-date review of peripheral actions and modification of parathyroid hormone. 74 refs.

Habener JF and Potts JT Jr.: Biosynthesis of parathyroid hormone. ***N Engl J Med*****, 299:580–585; 635–644; 1978.**
A complete review of this topic, including molecular aspects of parathyroid hormone (PTH) biosynthesis, general aspects of secretory protein synthesis, regulation of PTH secretion and clinical implications. 108 refs.

Treatment

Purnell DC, Scholz DA, Smith LH et al.: Treatment of primary hyperparathyroidism. ***Am J Med*****, 56:800–809, 1974.**
A review of treatment modalities available in primary hyperparathyroidism. Of 475 patients operated on, 78 percent had a single adenoma, 13 percent had multiple gland hyperplasia and 10 percent had negative explorations. The authors discuss what to do with this last group, and the medical management and follow-up of asymptomatic patients. 15 refs.

Davies DR: The surgery of primary hyperparathyroidism. ***Clin Endocrinol Metab*****, 3:253–265, 1974.**
A brief review of this topic. 11 refs.

Kaplan RA, Snyder WH, Stewart A and Pak CYC: Metabolic effects of parathyroidectomy in asymptomatic primary hyperparathyroidism. ***J Clin Endocrinol Metab*****, 42:415–426, 1976.**
Patients with either asymptomatic (six) or symptomatic (seven) primary hyperparathyroidism underwent parathyroidectomy. Operation corrected the decreased bone density, hypercalcemia and negative calcium balance, and reversed the decreased renal function in most patients. 26 refs.

Monchik JM, Doppman JL, Earll JM and Aurbach GD: Localizing of hyperfunctioning parathyroid tissue: Radioimmunoassay of parathyroid hormone on samples from the large veins of the neck and thorax and selectively catheterized thyroid veins. ***Am J Surg*****, 129:413–420, 1975.**
This difficult technique was used to evaluate 21 patients with hyperparathyroidism. Large vein sampling was not useful; the

authors claim correct localization in 14 of 17 patients who underwent selective venous sampling. 35 refs.

Evans TC Jr. and Edis AJ: High-resolution, real-time ultrasonography in the preoperative location of parathyroid tumors. ***N Engl J Med*, 301:532–534, 1979.**
The use of B-mode ultrasonography is described in the preoperative evaluation of 10 patients with hyperparathyroidism, thought to have large tumors because of severe hypercalcemia. Several successful tumor localizations are demonstrated; this technique may become very useful in the preoperative evaluation of primary hyperparathyroidism. 4 refs.

Wang CA: The anatomic basis of parathyroid surgery. ***Ann Surg*, 183:271–275, 1976.**
The anatomic location of parathyroid glands was established by neck dissection in 160 cadavers. Four patients had supernumerary glands, three with five and one with six. 6 refs.

Wang CA: Parathyroid re-exploration. A clinical and pathological study of 112 cases. ***Ann Surg*, 186:140–145, 1977.**
112 "second-look" operations for hyperparathyroidism are described, of which all but 10 were successful. Of 81 percent of parathyroids discovered in the neck, 38 percent were in the superior posterior mediastinum; of 19 percent in the mediastinum, 67 percent were in the upper anterior mediastinum. 10 refs.

Nathaniels EK, Nathaniels AM and Wang CA: Mediastinal parathyroid tumors: A clinical and pathologic study of 84 cases. ***Ann Surg*, 171:165–170, 1970.**
Of 400 patients with hyperparathyroidism, 84 had mediastinal tumors, 67 anterior and 17 posterior. The approach to these patients is discussed. 10 refs.

Wells SA Jr., Gunnells JC, Shelburne JD et al.: Transplantation of the parathyroid glands in man: Clinical indications and results. ***Surgery*, 78:34–44, 1975.**
29 patients underwent parathyroid transplantation, 28 autografts for secondary hyperparathyroidism or primary hyperplasia, and one allograft for hypoparathyroidism. Of 11 patients followed for 1 year, 10 were normocalcemic; graft function could be assessed by measuring PTH in the antecubital vein proximal to the graft. 15 refs.

Wells SA, Ellis GJ, Gunnells JC et al.: Parathyroid autotransplantation in primary parathyroid hyperplasia. ***N Engl J Med*, 295:57–62, 1976.**

Four patients with parathyroid hyperplasia underwent total parathyroidectomy and autotransplantation of tissue into the forearm. All patients were normocalcemic after 13 months; graft function could be assessed by antecubital venous sampling. (See also accompanying editorial.) 17 refs.

Parathyroid Carcinoma

Holmes EC, Morton DL and Ketcham AS: Parathyroid carcinoma: A collective review. *Ann Surg*, 169:631–640, 1969.
46 patients with parathyroid carcinoma are described. 60 percent were men; the age range was 12 to 72. All had symptoms and signs of severe hyperparathyroidism and hypercalcemia (average calcium 15.9 mg/dl). 50 percent of patients had a palpable mass; 50 percent had metastatic disease. 44 refs.

Schantz A and Castleman B: Parathyroid carcinoma. A study of 70 cases. *Cancer*, 31:600–605, 1973.
70 cases of parathyroid carcinoma are described. The average serum calcium was 15.2 mg/dl; most common signs and symptoms were bone disease, neck mass or kidney stones. The 5 year mortality appeared to be less than 50 percent. 9 refs.

Hypoparathyroidism

Breslau NA and Pak CYC: Hypoparathyroidism. *Metabolism*, 28:1,261–1,276, 1979.
A detailed, recent review of this syndrome, including the various variants of pseudohypoparathyroidism. 93 refs.

Nusynowitz ML, Frame B and Kolb FU: The spectrum of the hypoparathyroid states: A classification based on physiologic principles. *Medicine*, 55:105–119, 1976.
The authors attempt to classify hypocalcemic disorders on the basis of PTH levels, and describe complete differential diagnoses for "hormonopenic" and "hormonoplethoric" hypocalcemia. 114 refs.

Schneider AB and Sherwood LM: Pathogenesis and management of hypoparathyroidism and other hypocalcemic disorders. *Metabolism*, 24:871–898, 1975.
A detailed review of causes of hypocalcemia, with a short section on acute and chronic treatment. 131 refs.

Woodhouse NJY: Hypocalcemia and hypoparathyroidism. *Clin Endocrinol Metab*, 3:323–343, 1974.
A concise review of hypocalcemic and hypoparathyroid disorders, with emphasis on differential diagnosis and treatment. 93 refs.

Avioli LV: The therapeutic approach to hypoparathyroidism. ***Am J Med*, 57:34–42, 1974.**
The author briefly reviews the therapeutic approaches to hypoparathyroidism, chiefly with calcium and older vitamin D preparations. 103 refs.

Porter RH, Cox BG, Heaney D et al.: Treatment of hypoparathyroid patients with chlorthalidone. ***N Engl J Med*, 298:577–581, 1978.**
7 patients with idiopathic hypoparathyroidism were treated for up to 25 months with chlorthalidone and low salt diets, causing a significant increase in serum calcium and a decrease in urinary calcium excretion. This form of therapy may be effective in mild hypoparathyroidism. 36 refs.

Kooh SW, Fraser D, DeLuca HF et al.: Treatment of hypoparathyroidism and pseudohypoparathyroidism with metabolites of vitamin D: Evidence for impaired conversion of 25-hydroxyvitamin D to 1α, 25-dihydroxyvitamin D. ***N Engl J Med*, 293:840–844, 1975.**
In 2 children with hypoparathyroidism and 1 with pseudohypoparathyroidism, 100 times more 25-hydroxyvitamin D_3 than 1α, 25-hydroxyvitamin D_3 was needed to restore normocalcemia, suggesting a defect in renal hydroxylation of 25-hydroxyvitamin D_3 in these conditions. 30 refs.

Bell NH and Stern PH: Hypercalcemia and increases in serum hormone value during prolonged administration of 1α, 25-dihydroxyvitamin D. ***N Engl J Med*, 298:1,241–1,243, 1978.**
2 patients with pseudohypoparathyroidism were treated with oral 1α, 25-dihydroxyvitamin D. After six months of treatment they developed hypercalcemia, a possible side effect of this drug, which disappeared on cessation of treatment. 15 refs.

Mann JB, Alterman S and Hills AG: Albright's hereditary osteodystrophy comprising pseudohypoparathyroidism and pseudo-pseudohypoparathyroidism. ***Ann Intern Med*, 56:315–342, 1962.**
The authors describe a woman with pseudohypoparathyroidism and her son, who had pseudo-pseudohypoparathyroidism. They offer a complete review of the older literature. 73 refs.

Steinbach HL and Young DA: The roentgen appearance of pseudohypoparathyroidism (PH) and pseudo-pseudohypoparathyroidism (PPH). ***Am J Roentgenol*, 97:49–66, 1966.**
The radiographic manifestations of these two conditions are reviewed, and compared to other conditions in which short

fingers are found: brachyphalangia; peripheral dysostosis; chondro-ectodermal dysplasia; multiple familial exostosis and Turner's syndrome. 66 refs.

Farfel Z, Brickman AS, Kaslow HR et al.: Defect of receptor-cyclase coupling protein in pseudohypoparathyroidism, *N Engl J Med,* 303:237–242, 1980.
5 of 10 patients with pseudohypoparathyroidism had a deficiency in the activity of an adenyl-cyclase coupled protein from erythrocyte membranes necessary for cyclic AMP generation, possibly related to parathyroid hormone resistance in this condition. 32 refs.

Nusynowitz ML and Klein MH: Pseudoidiopathic hypoparathyroidism: Hypoparathyroidism with ineffective parathyroid hormone. *Am J Med,* 55:677–686, 1973.
One patient with this syndrome is described. It consists of hypocalcemia and elevated PTH levels, with normal renal responsiveness to exogenous PTH, indicating that the patient's endogenous PTH was defective. 39 refs.

Werder EA, Fischer JA, Illig R et al.: Pseudohypoparathyroidism and idiopathic hypoparathyroidism: Relationship between serum calcium and parathyroid hormone levels and urinary cyclic adenosine-3′,5′-monophosphate response to parathyroid extract. *J Clin Endocrinol Metab*, 47:872–879, 1978.
The authors evaluated 40 patients with hypocalcemia and/or pseudohypoparathyroidism. They were able to distinguish among hypoparathyroidism, pseudohypoparathyroidism types I and II and pseudo-pseudohypoparathyroidism on the basis of the above tests. 50 refs.

Rude RK, Oldham SB and Singer FR: Functional hypoparathyroidism and parathyroid hormone end-organ resistance in human magnesium deficiency. *Clin Endocrinol*, 5:209–224, 1976.
17 patients with hypocalcemia and severe hypomagnesemia were evaluated. Both impaired PTH secretion and end-organ resistance to PTH action were demonstrated. 60 refs.

Frame B, Hanson CA, Frost HM et al.: Renal resistance to parathyroid hormone with osteitis fibrosa, "pseudoparathyroidism." *Am J Med,* 52:311–321, 1972.
Two patients with renal but not skeletal resistance to parathyroid hormone are described. They had normal appearance, but hypocalcemia, hyperphosphatemia and osteitis fibrosa cystica. 22 refs.

Hypercalcemia (See Also Hyperparathyroidism)

General

Schneider AB and Sherwood LM: Calcium homeostasis and the pathogenesis and management of hypercalcemic disorders. ***Metabolism*****, 23:975–1,007, 1974.**
A lengthy review of the controls regulating the serum calcium concentration, and how these go haywire in hypercalcemic disorders. 171 refs.

Fraser P, Healy M, Rose N and Watson L: Discriminant functions in differential diagnosis of hypercalcemia. ***Lancet*****, 1:1,314–1,319, 1971.**
The authors describe a simple discriminant approach to the diagnosis of causes of hypercalcemia, which proved correct in 90 percent of 218 cases. 21 refs.

Skrabanek P, McPartlin J and Powell D: Tumor hypercalcemia and "ectopic hyperparathyroidism." ***Medicine*****, 59:262–282, 1980.**
An extensive, recent evaluation of the causes of the hypercalcemia of malignancy, in which data from 307 cases are discussed. The authors conclude that the evidence for ectopic PTH production by tumors is not well documented, and could find no single case where this was unequivocally present. 282 refs.

Buckle R: Ectopic PTH syndrome, pseudohyperparathyroidism; hypercalcemia of malignancy. ***Clin Endocrinol Metab*****, 3:237–251, 1974.**
A short review of this subject, with emphasis on the cause of the hypercalcemia. 32 refs.

Powell D, Singer FR, Murray TM et al.: Nonparathyroid humoral hypercalcemia in patients with neoplastic diseases. ***N Engl J Med*****, 289:176–181, 1973.**
9 of 11 patients with pseudohyperparathyroidism from tumors without bony metastases noted relief of hypercalcemia following removal or chemotherapy of their tumors. PTH was not detectable by radioimmunoassay in these patients, but tumor extracts caused bone resorbtion in vitro. 30 refs.

Muggia FM and Heinemann HO: Hypercalcemia associated with neoplastic disease. ***Ann Intern Med*****, 73:281–290, 1970.**
An early review of the common neoplastic causes of hypercalcemia. 91 refs.

Bockman RS: Hypercalcemia in malignancy. ***Clin Endocrinol Metab*****, 9:317–333, 1980.**
A brief, recent review, emphasizing recent theories on the pathogenesis of cancer-related hypercalcemia, with little discussion of treatment. 60 refs.

Lafferty FW: Pseudohyperparathyroidism. ***Medicine*****, 45:247–260, 1966.**
A detailed early review of the hypercalcemia of malignancy without bony metastases, in which 50 cases of this syndrome were compared to 17 cases of proven hyperparathyroidism. Hypernephroma and bronchogenic carcinoma accounted for 60 percent of the cases of pseudohyperparathyroidism. 109 refs.

Seyberth HW, Segre GV, Morgan JL et al.: Prostaglandins as mediators of hypercalcemia associated with certain types of cancer. ***N Engl J Med*****, 293:1,278–1,283, 1975.**
14 hypercalcemic patients with solid tumors had increased urinary levels of Prostaglandin E metabolites; aspirin or indomethacin decreased both urinary excretion of the metabolites and serum calcium in 6 of these patients. 35 refs.

Benson RC Jr., Riggs BL, Pickard BM and Arnaud CD: Radioimmunoassay of parathyroid hormone in hypercalcemic patients with malignant disease. ***Am J Med*****, 56:821–826, 1974.**
Of 108 hypercalcemic patients with cancer, 103 were found to have inappropriately elevated PTH levels, as determined by a C-terminal radioimmunoassay. Levels were similar in groups with and without obvious skeletal metastases. The authors maintain that ectopic PTH secretion causes hypercalcemia in malignancy. 25 refs.

Cushard WG, Simon AB, Canterbury JM and Reiss E: Parathyroid function in sarcoidosis. ***N Engl J Med*****, 286:395–398, 1972.**
In 26 unselected cases of sarcoidosis, 6 had hypercalcemia but 19 had undetectable levels of PTH, suggesting that most patients with sarcoidosis have functional hypoparathyroidism. 34 refs.

Goldstein RA, Israel HL, Becker KL and Moore CF: The infrequency of hypercalcemia in sarcoidosis. ***Am J Med*****, 51:21–30, 1971.**
Hypercalcemia was seen in only 8 of 364 patients (2.2 percent) with sarcoidosis, generally in patients with severe disease, suggesting that this complication is much less common than previously thought. 72 refs.

Winnacker JL, Becker KL and Katz S: Endocrine aspects of sarcoidosis. ***N Engl J Med*****, 278:427–434, 1968.**
A now dated review of hypercalcemia in sarcoidosis. 123 refs.

Stole RM, Smith LH, Wilson DM et al.: Hydrochlorothiazide effects on serum calcium and immunoreactive parathyroid hormone. ***Ann Intern Med*****, 77:587–591, 1972.**
9 normal subjects were treated with hydrochlorothiazide for 25 days; they developed higher total and ionized calcium concentrations during and for 2 weeks after therapy, without effect on PTH levels or protein binding of calcium. 28 refs.

Levine C, Greer RB III and Gordon SL: Hypercalcemia complicating fracture immobilization: A report of three cases. ***J Trauma*****, 15:70–72, 1975.**
A short report of three cases of immobilization hypercalcemia. The authors suggest that this entity may be much more common than is generally realized. 8 refs.

Marx SJ, Spiegel AM, Brown EM et al.: Divalent cation metabolism. Familial hypocalciuric hypercalcemia versus typical primary hyperparathyroidism. ***Am J Med*****, 65:235–242, 1978.**
When 23 patients with familial hypercalcemia were compared to 64 patients with hyperparathyroidism, the former group had higher creatinine clearance, higher serum magnesium levels and lower urinary excretion of calcium and magnesium, suggesting a difference in the renal handling of these cations. 28 refs.

Marx SJ, Spiegel AM, Brown EM and Aurbach GD: Family studies in patients with primary parathyroid hyperplasia. ***Am J Med*****, 62:698–706, 1977.**
Of 25 patients with primary parathyroid hyperplasia, 13 had some first degree relatives with hypercalcemia. Two autosomal dominant familial syndromes could be separated: familial hypocalciuric hypercalcemia and multiple endocrine neoplasia Type I. Distinctions between the two groups are discussed. 42 refs.

Foley TP, Harrison HC, Arnaud CD and Harrison HE: Familial benign hypercalcemia. ***J Pediatr*****, 81:1,060–1,067, 1972.**
A syndrome is described of benign familial hypercalcemia with normal PTH levels and an autosomal dominant inheritance in 11 members of 1 extended family. 32 refs.

Bronsky D, Dubin A, Waldstein SS and Kushner DS: Calcium and electrocardiogram (Parts I-III). ***Am J Cardiol*****, 7:840–843, 1961.**

A detailed review of this subject, based on the study of 22 patients with hypoparathyroidism, and 33 patients with hypercalcemia of various causes. In general, the Q-T interval was inversely proportional to the serum calcium level, except at very high calcium concentrations. 52 refs.

Walsh FB and Howard JE: Conjunctival and corneal lesions in hypercalcemia. ***J Clin Endocrinol Metab,*** **7:644–652, 1947.**
A classic article describing two types of eye lesions in hypercalcemia: band keratitis and conjunctival crystals (probably calcium phosphate). The authors found one of these lesions in nearly half the patients with hypercalcemia they evaluated. 3 refs.

Treatment

Deflos LJ and Neer R: Medical management of the hypercalcemia of malignancy. ***Ann Rev Med,*** **25:323–331, 1974.**
A brief review of the postulated mechanisms of hypercalcemia in malignancy and the various treatments, including hydration, diuretics, inorganic phosphate, mithramycin, steroids, calcitonin and dialysis. 40 refs.

Goldsmith RS: Treatment of hypercalcemia. ***Med Clin North Am,*** **56:951–960, 1972.**
A brief and concise review of available treatments for acute hypercalcemia. 12 refs.

Suki WN, Yium JJ, VonMinden M et al.: Acute treatment of hypercalcemia with furosemide. ***N Engl J Med,*** **283:836–840, 1970.**
Eight patients with moderate to severe hypercalcemia were treated with large doses of furosemide with water and electrolyte replacement; six patients achieved near normal calciums through increased urinary calcium excretion. This therapy is compared to other standard treatments. 22 refs.

Slayton RE, Shnider BI, Elias E et al.: New approach to the treatment of hypercalcemia. The effect of short-term treatment with mithramycin. ***Clin Pharmacol Ther,*** **12:833–837, 1971.**
Mithramycin (25 μg/kg body weight as a single intravenous injection) was given after hydration to 89 patients with hypercalcemia of malignancy, of which 69 qualified for inclusion in the study. Complete normalization of serum calcium was achieved on 56 of 92 occasions; 6 patients failed to respond. Five consecutive daily doses appeared to be safe. 16 refs.

Perlia CP, Gubisch NJ, Wolter S et al.: Mithramycin treatment of hypercalcemia. ***Cancer,*** **25:389–394, 1970.**

32 patients with hypercalcemia of malignancy were treated with mithramycin (25 μg/kg body weight as a single intravenous injection). Prompt decreases in serum calcium levels were seen in all patients. 30 refs.

Fulmer DH, Dimich AB, Rothschild EO and Laird Myers WP: Treatment of hypercalcemia. Comparison of intravenously administered phosphate, sulfate and hydrocortisone. ***Arch Intern Med,*** **129:923–930, 1972.**
Intravenous phosphate infusions were markedly superior to intravenous sulfate or hydrocortisone in reducing serum calcium levels in 22 patients with the hypercalcemia of malignancy. The calcium decrease correlated with the amount of phosphate infused. 9 of 20 courses were associated with an increase in BUN. 27 refs.

Massry SG, Mueller E, Silverman AG and Kleeman CR: Inorganic phosphate treatment of hypercalcemia. ***Arch Intern Med,*** **121:309–312, 1968.**
18 patients with hypercalcemia received either oral or intravenous phosphate. Renal microscopic calcification was noted in two patients, but all experienced a decrease in serum calcium concentrations. Few other side effects were noted in this study. 16 refs.

Carey RW, Schmitt GW, Kopald HH et al.: Massive extraskeletal calcification during phosphate treatment of hypercalcemia. ***Arch Intern Med,*** **122:150–155, 1968.**
A case report of a patient with disseminated carcinoma and hypercalcemia who developed extensive metastatic calcification during phosphate therapy. 18 refs.

Shackney S and Hasson J: Precipitous fall in serum calcium, hypotension and acute renal failure after intravenous phosphate therapy for hypercalcemia. Report of two cases. ***Ann Intern Med,*** **66:906–916, 1967.**
Two cases of renal failure and hypotension that developed after intravenous phosphate treatment of hypercalcemia are described. One patient had diffuse metastatic calcification of many tissues. The authors discuss the hazards of this type of therapy. 47 refs.

Silva OL and Becker KL: Salmon calcitonin in the treatment of hypercalcemia. ***Arch Intern Med,*** **132:337–339, 1973.**
Of 23 patients with hypercalcemia treated with calcitonin, 17 experienced decreases in serum calcium concentrations. The response was generally only partial; six patients did not respond. Side effects were rare. 11 refs.

Strauch BS and Ball MF: Hemodialysis in the treatment of severe hypercalcemia. ***JAMA*****, 235:1,347–1,348, 1976.**
A single patient with life-threatening hypercalcemia (serum concentration 21 mg/dl) was treated with hemodialysis before removal of a large parathyroid adenoma. Serum calcium decreased about one mg/dl/hr while the patient was being dialyzed. 10 refs.

Osteoporosis (See Also Estrogen Therapy)

Wheeler M: Osteoporosis. ***Med Clin North Am*****, 60:1,213–1,224, 1976.**
A short, general overview of the whole problem of osteopenia. 16 refs.

Thomson DL and Frame B: Involutional osteopenia: Current concepts. ***Ann Intern Med,*** **85:789–803, 1976.**
An excellent recent review of diagnostic tests and recent therapeutic trials in patients with osteoporosis. 173 refs.

Avioli LV: Senile and postmenopausal osteoporosis. ***Adv Intern Med,*** **21:391–415, 1976.**
A thorough review of this syndrome, with a good bibliography of the older literature. 164 refs.

Nordin BEC: Clinical significance and pathogenesis of osteoporosis. ***Br Med J*****, 1:571–576, 1971.**
A brief but thorough review of the etiologies and pathogenesis of osteoporosis. 44 refs.

Gallagher JC, Aaron J, Horsman A et al.: The crush fracture syndrome in postmenopausal women. ***Clin Endocrinol Metab,*** **2:293–315, 1973.**
A detailed analysis of this syndrome, a common presentation of osteoporosis, in a series of 58 patients. All were postmenopausal women. 20 refs.

Teitelbaum SL, Rosenberg EM, Richardson CA and Avioli LV: Histological studies of bone from normocalcemic postmenopausal osteoporotic patients with increased circulating parathyroid hormone. ***J Clin Endocrinol Metab,*** **42:537–543, 1976.**
Of 16 postmenopausal women with osteoporosis, 6 had elevated PTH levels as well as increased cortical osteoclast counts on bone biopsy. The authors suggest that postmenopausal osteoporosis may be a heterogeneous disorder. 25 refs.

Hahn TJ: Corticosteroid-induced osteopenia. ***Arch Intern Med,*** **138:882–885, 1978.**

A short, recent review of this extremely troublesome disorder, with tentative suggestions on prevention. 38 refs.

Gallagher JC, Aaron J, Horsman A et al.: Corticosteroid osteoporosis. *Clin Endocrinol Metab,* 2:355–368, 1973.
A brief review of this extremely important and common form of osteopenia. 32 refs.

Cryer PE and Kissane JM: Osteopenia. *Am J Med,* 69:915–922, 1980.
This clinicopathologic conference reviewed a case of osteopenia associated with systemic mastocytosis. Other metabolic causes of osteopenia were also reviewed. 15 refs.

Griffith GC, Nichols G Jr., Asher JD and Flanagan B: Heparin osteoporosis. *JAMA*, 193:91–94, 1965.
10 of 117 patients received more than 15,000 units of heparin per day for longer than 6 months; 6 of these 10 developed spontaneous spine or rib fractures. No fractures occurred in 107 patients on lower dose, long-term therapy. 15 refs.

Gordan GS: Drug treatment of the osteoporoses. *Ann Rev Pharmacol Toxicol*, 18:253–268, 1978.
An extensive, recent review of therapies for postmenopausal, corticosteroid-induced and immobilization osteopenia. 104 refs.

Lindsay R, Hart DM, Aitken JM et al.: Long-term prevention of postmenopausal osteoporosis by oestrogen. *Lancet,* 1:1,038–1,041, 1976.
Estrogen treatment of 63 women after oophorectomy for 5 years resulted in a decrease in bone mineral density of 0.4 percent/year, compared with 2.7 percent/year in 57 placebo treated women. 21 refs.

Horsman A, Gallagher JC, Simpson M and Nordin BEC: Prospective trial of oestrogen and calcium in postmenopausal women. *Br Med J*, 2:789–792, 1977.
Postmenopausal women (72) were treated with calcium, estrogen or not treated. Estrogen treatment prevented the bone loss (evaluated by densitometry and morphometry) observed in the controls; calcium retarded it less effectively. 11 refs.

Recker RR, Saville PD and Heaney RP: Effect of estrogens and calcium carbonate on bone loss in postmenopausal women. *Ann Intern Med*, 87:649–655, 1977.
60 postmenopausal women were treated with estrogen plus testosterone, calcium carbonate or not treated, and were followed for 2 years. Bone density decreased by 2.88 percent/

year in the control group, 1.83 percent/year in the calcium group and 0.73 percent/year in the hormone group. 48 refs.

Lindsay R, Hart, DM, MacLean A et al.: Bone response to termination of oestrogen treatment. ***Lancet*****, 1:1,325–1,327, 1978.**
Of 43 patients with postmenopausal osteoporosis followed for 8 years, 15 took estrogens and did not lose bone, whereas patients treated with placebo (14) lost a significant amount. Estrogens were discontinued after 4 years in 14 patients; their bone mineral then decreased at a mean rate of 2.5 percent/year. 10 refs.

Jowsey J, Riggs BL, Kelly PJ and Hoffman DL: Effect of combined therapy with sodium fluoride, vitamin D and calcium in osteoporosis. ***Am J Med*****, 53:43–49, 1972.**
11 patients with osteoporosis were treated with the above combination therapy for 1 year. Bone biopsy data suggested that optimal doses of each drug in these combinations could restore bone mass in osteoporosis. 46 refs.

Osteomalacia

Frame B and Parfitt AM: Osteomalacia: Current concepts. ***Ann Intern Med*****, 89:966–982, 1978.**
An excellent, comprehensive and recent review, focusing on newer forms of treatment with metabolites of vitamin D. 133 refs.

Habener JF and Mahaffey JE: Osteomalacia and disorders of vitamin D metabolism. ***Ann Rev Med*****, 29:327–342, 1978.**
A brief, recent review of the various osteomalacic syndromes. 72 refs.

Mankin HJ: Rickets, osteomalacia and renal osteodystrophy. ***J Bone Joint Surg*****, 56A:101–128, 352–386, 1974.**
A complete, detailed review of these syndromes, with an interesting historical review and many helpful radiographs. 233 refs.; 387 refs.

Hahn TJ and Avioli LV: Anticonvulsant osteomalacia. ***Arch Intern Med*****, 135:997–1,000, 1975.**
A brief review of this entity based on a single case report; the first author discusses therapeutic and prophylactic vitamin D administration. 12 refs.

Hahn TJ, Hendin BA, Scharp CR et al.: Serum 25-hydroxycalciferol levels and bone mass in children on chronic anticonvulsant therapy. ***N Engl J Med*****, 292:550–554, 1975.**

Serum calcium, 25-hydroxycalciferol and bone mineral density were decreased in 56 children on chronic anticonvulsant therapy compared to 51 controls. The authors concluded that prophylactic vitamin D administration was warranted in these patients. 28 refs.

Avioli LV, Birge SJ and Lee SW: Effects of prednisone on vitamin D metabolism in man. ***J Clin Endocrinol*, 28:1,341–1,346, 1968.**
Prednisone administration to four normal subjects caused increased vitamin D_3 turnover and a decreased production of a biologically active metabolite, leading to decreased gut absorbtion of calcium. 35 refs.

Sitrin M, Meredith S and Rosenberg IH: Vitamin D deficiency and bone disease in gastrointestinal disorders. ***Arch Intern Med*, 138:886–888, 1978.**
A very brief but current review of these relatively common causes of osteomalacia. 32 refs.

Brooks MH, Bell NH, Love L et al.: Vitamin D-dependent rickets type II: Resistance of target organs to 1,25-dihydroxyvitamin D. ***N Engl J Med*, 298:996–999, 1978.**
One patient is described with hypocalcemia, hyperparathyroidism, osteomalacia and abnormally elevated serum 1,25-dihydroxyvitamin D, who responded to vitamin D_3. The authors propose that she had a new syndrome of peripheral target organ resistance to 1,25-dihydroxy vitamin D. 23 refs.

Fraser D, Kooh SW, Kind HP et al.: Pathogenesis of hereditary vitamin D-dependent rickets: An inborn error of vitamin D metabolism involving defective conversion of 25-hydroxyvitamin D to 1α,25-dihydroxyvitamin D. ***N Engl J Med*, 289:817–822, 1973.**
In 5 patients with vitamin D-dependent rickets, relatively small doses of 1,25-dihydroxyvitamin D were required to heal bone lesions, whereas massive doses of several precursors of this metabolite were ineffective. 45 refs.

Fraser D and Scriver CR: Familial forms of vitamin D-resistant rickets revisited. X-linked hypophosphatemia and autosomal recessive vitamin D-dependency. ***Am J Clin Nutr*, 29:1,315–1,329, 1976.**
These two types of "vitamin D-resistant" rickets are reviewed, with comments on their treatment with modern vitamin D metabolites. 102 refs.

Fitzgerald F: Clinical hypophosphatemia. ***Ann Rev Med,*** **29:177–189, 1978.**
A brief, recent review of hypophosphatemia. 76 refs.

Knochel JP: The pathophysiology and clinical characteristics of severe hypophosphatemia. ***Arch Intern Med,*** **137:203–220, 1977.**
A detailed review of phosphate-depletion syndromes in man, with emphasis on the metabolic effects of profound hypophosphatemia. 162 refs.

Lotz M, Zisman E and Bartter FC: Evidence for a phosphorus-depletion syndrome in man. ***N Engl J Med,*** **278:409–414, 1968.**
Prolonged treatment of three normal subjects and three with parathyroid disorders with phosphorus-binding antacids produced hypophosphatemia, increased intestinal calcium absorption, hypocalciuria, increased bone resorbtion and marked physical debility. 47 refs.

Parfitt AM and Frame B: Treatment of rickets and osteomalacia. ***Semin Drug Treat,*** **2:83-115, 1972.**
An extensive review of the diagnosis and treatment of rickets and osteomalacia, using analytical methods and vitamin D analogues available in 1972. 256 refs.

Glorieux FH, Scriver CR, Reade TM et al.: Use of phosphate and vitamin D to prevent dwarfism and rickets in X-linked hypophosphatemia. ***N Engl J Med,*** **287:481–487, 1972.**
Phosphate and vitamin D therapy in eight children with the above disorder resulted in increased serum phosphorus concentrations, decreased x-ray evidence of rickets and increased growth, without ectopic calcification. 56 refs.

Renal Osteodystrophy

Stanbury SW: Azotaemic renal osteodystrophy. ***Clin Endocrinol Metab,*** **1:267–304, 1972.**
A long, complete but somewhat dated review of this complex topic, with emphasis on the disordered state of vitamin D and PTH metabolism. About 160 refs.

Alvarez-Ude F, Feest TG, Ward MK et al.: Hemodialysis bone disease: Correlation between clinical, histologic and other findings. ***Kidney Int,*** **14:68-73, 1978.**
Studies of 85 patients on chronic dialysis revealed bone pain in 44 percent, histologic osteomalacia in 71 percent and osteitis fibrosa in 80 percent. Pain was correlated with osteomalacia but not with osteitis fibrosa. 30 refs.

Goldsmith RS, Johnson WJ and Arnaud CD: The hyperparathyroidism of renal failure: Pathophysiology and treatment. ***Clin Endocrinol Metab*****, 3:305–321, 1974.**
A brief review of renal bone disease, with sections on pathophysiology, therapy and transplantation. 58 refs.

Massry SG, Coburn JW, Popovtzer MM et al.: Secondary hyperparathyroidism in chronic renal failure. The clinical spectrum in uremia, during hemodialysis and after renal transplantation. ***Arch Intern Med*****, 124:431–441, 1969.**
An interesting clinical description of 15 patients with secondary hyperparathyroidism and 27 controls with comparable renal failure. The clinical, laboratory and x-ray findings of secondary hyperparathyroidism are reviewed. 31 refs.

Ibels LS, Alfrey AC, Huffer WE and Weil R III: Aseptic necrosis of bone following renal transplantation: Experience in 194 transplant recipients and review of the literature. ***Medicine*****, 57:25–45, 1978.**
Of 194 renal transplant patients, mostly on prednisone, 40 (21 percent) developed symptomatic avascular necrosis of bone, in which 101 joints were affected. Joint pain was the usual presenting symptom. 102 refs.

David DS: Calcium metabolism in renal failure. ***Am J Med*****, 58:48–56, 1975.**
A concise review of the effects renal failure has on various aspects of calcium metabolism. 50 refs.

Freitag J, Martin KJ, Hruska KA et al.: Impaired parathyroid hormone metabolism in patients with chronic renal failure. ***N Engl J Med*****, 298:29–32, 1978.**
The authors measured PTH in a total of 217 patients with various parathyroid and renal disorders. Levels of PTH as measured by the C-terminal immunoassay were 50-fold higher than normal in anephric patients on dialysis. The renal clearance of PTH should be kept in mind when assessing secondary hyperparathyroidism. 15 refs.

Malluche HH, Goldstein DA and Massry SG: Osteomalacia and hyperparathyroid bone disease in patients with nephrotic syndrome. ***J Clin Invest*****, 63:494–500, 1979.**
6 patients with nephrotic syndrome but normal renal function had low serum 25-hydroxyvitamin D levels, low to normal serum calcium, elevated serum PTH and histologic evidence of osteomalacia; this represents a new type of "renal osteodystrophy." 17 refs.

Fournier A, Bordier P, Gueris J et al.: Comparison of 1 α-hydroxycholecalciferol and 25-hydroxycholecalciferol in the treatment of renal osteodystrophy: Greater effect of 25-hydroxycholecalciferol on bone mineralization. ***Kidney Int,*** **15:196–204, 1979.**
Treatment with 1 of the above 2 vitamin D derivatives was attempted in 10 uremic patients on dialysis. The authors concluded that large doses of 25-hydroxycholecalciferol cause more bone remineralization, but may cause more severe hypercalcemia than the 1α derivative. 38 refs.

Recker R, Schoenfeld P, Letteri J et al.: The efficacy of calcifediol in renal osteodystrophy. ***Arch Intern Med,*** **138:857–863, 1978.**
63 patients on chronic dialysis were treated with 25-hydroxycholecalciferol (calcifediol). Clinical bone pain and serum alkaline phosphatase improved in most patients. 39 refs.

Ahmed KY, Varghese Z, Wills MR et al.: Long-term effects of small doses of 1,25-dihydroxycholecalciferol in renal osteodystrophy. ***Lancet,*** **1:629–632, 1978.**
5 patients with renal osteodystrophy were treated with the above metabolite and calcium for 4 to 16 months. Intestinal calcium absorbtion became normal, plasma alkaline phosphatase and PTH decreased, and bone mineralization increased. 12 refs.

Bordier P, Zingraff J, Gueris J et al.: The effect of 1α $(OH)D_3$ and 1α,25$(OH)_2D_3$ on the bone in patients with renal osteodystrophy. ***Am J Med,*** **64:101–107, 1978.**
In six patients with renal osteodystrophy treated for three weeks each with the above compounds, serum calcium and PTH levels tended to normalize, whereas the alkaline phosphatase activity and osteoid volume did not change. This study provides additional evidence that vitamin D metabolites cannot completely correct the bone disease of chronic renal failure. 31 refs.

Brickman AS, Sherrard DJ, Jowsey J et al.: 1,25-dihydroxycholecalciferol. Effect on skeletal lesions and plasma parathyroid hormone levels in uremic osteodystrophy. ***Arch Intern Med,*** **134:883–888, 1974.**
8 patients with uremic osteodystrophy were treated with 1,25-dihydroxycholecalciferol for 8 to 17 weeks. Serum calcium levels increased slightly, serum PTH decreased in six and biopsy appearance improved in several patients. 31 refs.

Paget's Disease of Bone

Krane SM: Paget's disease of bone. ***Clin Orthop*****, 127:24–36, 1977.**
A concise recent review of Paget's disease, including its epidemiology, histology, metabolic and biochemical features, clinical findings and modern approach to therapy. 81 refs.

Nagant de Deuxchaisnes C and Krane SM: Paget's disease of bone: Clinical and metabolic observations. ***Medicine*****, 43:233–266, 1964.**
A complete and detailed review of the earlier literature on Paget's disease. 262 refs.

Doyle FH, Pennock J, Greenberg PB et al.: Radiological evidence of a dose-related response to long-term treatment of Paget's disease with human calcitonin. ***Br J Radiol*****, 47:1–8, 1974.**
28 patients with symptomatic Paget's disease were treated with synthetic human calcitonin for 10 to 40 months. 1 weekly injection of .5 mg was ineffective; increasing doses correlated with increasing frequency of radiologic and symptomatic improvement. 6 refs.

DeRose J, Singer FR, Avramides A et al.: Response of Paget's disease to porcine and salmon calcitonins. Effects of long-term treatment. ***Am J Med,*** **56:858–866, 1974.**
Patients (49) with Paget's were treated for 4 to 41 months with porcine or synthetic salmon calcitonin. 75 percent experienced relief of pain and neurologic defects; 20 percent experienced nausea or rash. Binding antibodies to both calcitonins were common, but were not responsible for disease "rebound." 16 refs.

Avramides A, Flores A, DeRose J and Wallach S: Paget's disease of the bone: Observations after cessation of long-term synthetic salmon calcitonin treatment. ***J Clin Endocrinol Metab,*** **42:459–463, 1976.**
13 patients with Paget's were treated for an average of 22 months with calcitonin, then followed for a year after its discontinuation. Symptoms continued improved in 10; they recurred in 3. Alkaline phosphatase increased to pretreatment levels by six months. 24 refs.

Canfield R, Rosner W, Skinner J et al.: Diphosphonate therapy of Paget's disease of bone. ***J Clin Endocrinol Metab,*** **44:96–106, 1977.**
The effect of EHDP in different doses on Paget's disease was assessed in 75 patients in a controlled, randomized, double-

blind protocol. The optimum dose appeared to be 5 mg EHDP/kg/day. 30 refs.

Russell RGG, Smith R, Preston C et al.: Diphosphonates in Paget's disease. ***Lancet,*** **1:894–898, 1974.**
47 patients with Paget's disease were treated with sodium etidronate (EHDP) for up to 6 months. Decreases in alkaline phosphatase were dose related; clinical remissions lasted long after the drug was discontinued. No fractures or other serious side effects were noted. 26 refs.

Khairi MRA, Johnston CC, Altman RD et al.: Treatment of Paget's disease of bone (osteitis deformans). Results of a one-year study with sodium etidronate. ***JAMA,*** **230:562–567, 1974.**
50 symptomatic patients with Paget's were treated with sodium etidronate (EHDP) or placebo, with a "cross over" at 6 months. EHDP clearly caused decreases in alkaline phosphatase and symptoms; the benefit was dose related and persisted after discontinuing the drug. 23 refs.

Lebbin D, Ryan WG and Schwarz TB.: Outpatient treatment of Paget's disease of bone with mithramycin. ***Ann Intern Med,*** **81:635–637, 1974.**
13 patients with severe, widespread Paget's were treated with mithramycin on 2 schedules. All experienced a decrease in pain and alkaline phosphatase; toxicity was transient and reversible if the drug was stopped. 6 refs.

DISORDERS OF THE ENDOCRINE PANCREAS AND RELATED DISORDERS

Physiology, Diagnosis and Genetic Aspects

National Diabetes Data Group: Classification and diagnosis of diabetes mellitus and other categories of glucose intolerance. ***Diabetes,*** **28:1,039–1,057, 1979.**
New international guidelines are presented for the diagnosis of diabetes, with a new classification based on insulin dependence or independence, obesity and occurrence during gestation. 67 refs.

Sherwin R and Felig P: Pathophysiology of diabetes mellitus. ***Med Clin North Am,*** **62:695–711, 1978.**
A readable review of the effects of diabetes on metabolic processes. 67 refs.

Pfeifer MA, Halter JB and Porte D Jr: Insulin secretion in diabetes mellitus. ***Am J Med,*** **70:579–588, 1981.**

The authors review normal insulin secretion, and propose an interesting model of β-cell dysfunction in Type II diabetes. The model explains how the β-cells and peripheral tissues interact in this disease; it remains to be proven. 53 refs.

Reaven GM: Insulin-independent diabetes mellitus: Metabolic characteristics. ***Metabolism*, 29:445–454, 1980.**
A brief, recent review of the metabolic abnormalities associated with various grades of Type II (adult-onset) diabetes. 42 refs.

Olefsky JM and Kolterman OG: Mechanisms of insulin resistance in obesity and noninsulin-dependent (Type II) diabetes. ***Am J Med*, 70:151–168, 1981.**
A recent review of this complex topic. 59 refs.

Unger RH, Dobbs RE and Orci L: Insulin, glucagon and somatostatin in the regulation of metabolism. ***Ann Rev Physiol*, 40:307–343, 1978.**
A review of recent anatomic and functional information on pancreatic endocrine cells and their secretions. 176 refs.

Cahill GF Jr.: Physiology of insulin in man. ***Diabetes*, 20:785–799, 1971.**
A classic review of insulin action and related metabolic actions in man, before insulin receptors came into vogue. 56 refs.

Ashcroft SJH: Glucoreceptor mechanisms and the control of release and biosynthesis. ***Diabetologia*, 18:5–15, 1980.**
A review of what is known about the interactions between stimulus and secretion of pancreatic insulin. 81 refs.

Davidson MB: The effect of aging on carbohydrate metabolism: A review of the English literature and a practical approach to the diagnosis of diabetes mellitus in the elderly. ***Metabolism*, 28:688–705, 1979.**
The author evaluates the data indicating impaired glucose tolerance in the elderly, and discusses several theories of its pathogenesis. 705 refs.

Felig P, Wahren J, Sherwin R and Hendler R: Insulin, glucagon and somatostatin in normal physiology and diabetes mellitus. ***Diabetes*, 25:1,091–1,099, 1976.**
Recent studies on insulin-glucagon relationships are reviewed; the authors conclude that insulin deficiency is the primary problem in diabetes, with glucagon playing a subsidiary role in both physiology and pathology. 43 refs.

Czech MP: Insulin action and the regulation of hexose transport. ***Diabetes*, 29:399–409, 1980.**

A brief review of recent information of the nature of the insulin receptor and its relationship to the hexose transport mechanism. 141 refs.

Barnett AH, Eff C, Leslie RDG and Pyke DA: Diabetes in identical twins. A study of 200 pairs. *Diabetologia*, 20:87–93, 1981.
In an update of their previous twin studies, the authors found that twins were concordant for diabetes in 54% of 147 pairs where one twin had Type I diabetes, but in 91% of 53 pairs where one twin had Type II diabetes. 16 refs.

Rotter JI and Rimoin DL: The genetics of the glucose intolerance disorders. *Am J Med*, 70:116–126, 1981.
The authors review the current information on the inheritance of various types of diabetes, and conclude that there is a great deal of genetic heterogeneity, even within groups thought to be relatively homogeneous, e.g., maturity-onset diabetes of the young. 73 refs.

Neel JV The genetics of juvenile-onset type diabetes mellitus. *N Engl J Med*, 297:1,062–1,063, 1977.
A brief, skeptical review of recent literature. 13 refs.

Rubinstein P, Sucin-Foca N and Nicholson JF: Genetics of juvenile diabetes mellitus. A recessive gene closely linked to HLA-D and with 50 percent penetrance. *N Engl J Med*, 297:1,036–1,040, 1977.
Studies of 31 families with 1 or more diabetic children purported to show a "diabetes-predisposing" gene linked to HLA-D with about 50 percent penetrance. (See also accompanying editorial.) 35 refs.

Cudworth AG and Woodrow JC: HL-A system and diabetes mellitus. *Diabetes*, 24:345–349, 1975.
New data from 100 diabetic patients were used to determine a positive association of diabetes with HL-A antigens HL-A8 and W15. 22 refs.

Nelson PG, Pyke DA, Cudworth AG et al.: Histocompatibility antigens in diabetic identical twins. *Lancet*, II:193–194, 1975.
These authors did histocompatibility typing on 84 pairs of diabetic identical twins, 22 with maturity-onset and 62 with at least one twin having juvenile-onset diabetes (31 pairs were discordant, 31 concordant). The frequency of the W15 antigen was similar in concordant and discordant pairs, while HL-A8 was increased only in the concordant pairs. These data suggest two different alleles controlling genetic susceptility to diabetes. 13 refs.

Daily Management of Diabetes

Galloway JA and Bressler R: Insulin treatment in diabetes. ***Med Clin North Am,*** **62:663–680, 1978.**
An informative recent review of insulin pharmacology and problems with its clinical use. 76 refs.

Guerra SMO and Kitabchi AE: Comparison of the effectiveness of various routes of insulin injection: Insulin levels and glucose response in normal subjects. ***J Clin Endocrinol Metab,*** **42:869–874, 1976.**
Insulin injected by various routes in 14 lean nondiabetic subjects caused higher blood insulin levels and more rapid and deeper blood glucose decreases in this order: intravenous, intramuscular and subcutaneous. 24 refs.

Koivisto VA and Felig P: Alterations in insulin absorbtion and blood glucose control associated with varying insulin injection sites in diabetic patients. ***Ann Intern Med,*** **92:59–61, 1980.**
In seven diabetic patients, radioactive insulin disappeared from the abdominal wall much faster than from the arm or leg; absorption from the arm was 40 percent greater than from the leg. The authors recommend staying in one anatomic region to minimize variations in insulin absorbtion. 16 refs.

Arky RA: Current principles of dietary therapy of diabetes mellitus. ***Med Clin North Am,*** **62:655–662, 1978.**
A short, sensible review on the dietary management of diabetes, emphasizing hypocaloric diets for obese patients and regularly spaced meals for insulin-requiring juvenile-onset patients. 32 refs.

Ensinck JW and Bierman EL: Dietary management of diabetes mellitus. ***Ann Rev Med,*** **30:155–170, 1979.**
A brief review of traditional diabetic dietary teachings, with a short discussion of the possible relationship between diet and atherosclerosis. 56 refs.

Bierman EL, Albrink MJ, Arky RA et al.: Principles of nutrition and dietary recommendations for patients with diabetes mellitus: 1971. ***Diabetes,*** **20:633–634, 1971.**
This short policy statement of the American Diabetes Association recommends weight loss in obese diabetics and regularity of food intake in insulin-requiring diabetics, and ". . . there no longer appears to be any need to restrict disproportionately the intake of carbohydrates in the diet of most diabetic patients." No refs.

West KM: Diet therapy of diabetes: An analysis of failure. ***Ann Intern Med,*** **79:425–434, 1973.**

A complete appraisal of diet in diabetes and an analysis of common cause of dietary failures. The author also emphasizes the differences in dietary treatment of obese, noninsulin-requiring patients and lean, insulin-requiring patients. 79 refs.

Bunn HF: Evaluation of glycosylated hemoglobin in diabetic patients. ***Diabetes*****, 30:613–617, 1981.**
The author reviews the chemistry of glycosylated hemoglobins, and their utility as an index of glycemic control in diabetics. 67 refs.

Tattersall R and Gale E: Patient self-monitoring of blood glucose and refinements of conventional insulin treatment. ***Am J Med*****, 70:177–182, 1981.**
The authors review recent data about home monitoring of blood glucose and conclude that this technique is most useful for patients with brittle diabetes, pregnancy, abnormal renal thresholds, nocturnal hypoglycemia or those attempting "super" control for various reasons. 30 refs.

Rizza RA, Gerich JE, Haymond MW et al: Control of blood sugar in insulin-dependent diabetes: Comparison of an artificial endocrine pancreas, continuous subcutaneous insulin infusion, and intensified conventional insulin therapy. ***N Engl J Med*****, 303:1313–1318, 1980.**
Six patients with Type I diabetes underwent insulin delivery by means of a closed-loop system, open-loop infusion, or intensive conventional (injection) therapy in a clinical research center setting. There was no difference in the glycemic control achieved by the three regimens; glycemic profiles from non-diabetic patients were superior. 29 refs.

Soeldner JS: Treatment of diabetes mellitus by devices. ***Am J Med*****, 70:183–194, 1981.**
A recent review of this topic, with emphasis on the instrumentation employed. 65 refs.

Sutherland DER: Pancreas and islet transplantation. II. Clinical trials. ***Diabetologia*****, 20:435–450, 1981.**
The author reviews the current status of islet and pancreatic transplantation in man with detailed explanations of technique. 403 refs.

Complications of Diabetes

General

Raskin P: Diabetic regulation and its relationship to microangiopathy. ***Metabolism*****, 27:235–252, 1978.**

Recent review of this complicated question with emphasis on renal pathology; of course, the evidence for good control is still not complete. 73 refs.

Tchobroutsky G: Relation of diabetic control to development of microvascular complications. *Diabetologia,* 15:143–152, 1978.
Good review summarizing recent evidence in favor of tight control of blood glucose. 148 refs.

Pirart J: Diabetes mellitus and its degenerative complications: A prospective study of 4,400 patients observed between 1947 and 1973. *Diabetes Care,* 1:168–188; 252–263, 1978.
An ambitious prospective study by two dedicated Belgians, the best demonstration to date of the natural history of diabetic complications. In their hands, good "control" decreased the prevalence of nephropathy, neuropathy and retinopathy, but not leg or coronary atherosclerosis. Also included is a complete literature review. 208 refs.

Siperstein MD, Foster DW, Knowles HC Jr. et al.: Control of blood glucose and diabetic vascular disease. *N Engl J Med,* 296:1,060–1,063, 1977.
A brief editorial pointing out the hazards of "tight" blood glucose control, emphasizing that it has not been shown to affect the development of diabetic angiopathy. 31 refs.

Cahill GF Jr., Etzwiler DD and Freinkel N: "Control" and diabetes. *N Engl J Med,* 294:1,004–1,005, 1976.
A brief editorial stating the policy of The American Diabetes Association on control of blood glucose: ". . . the weight of evidence . . . strongly supports the concept that the microvascular complications of diabetes are decreased by reduction of blood glucose concentrations." 15 refs.

McMillan DE and Ditzel J, Eds.: Proceedings of a conference on diabetic microangiopathy. *Diabetes,* 25:suppl. 2, 805–930, 1976.
22 papers on diabétic microangiopathy are included in this symposium, with emphasis on the histological and biochemical findings.

Kaplan MH and Feinstein AR: A critique of methods in reported studies of long-term vascular complications in patients with diabetes mellitus. *Diabetes,* 22:160–174, 1973.
These authors critically evaluated 33 papers dealing with vascular complications of diabetes, and found methodologic problems in all. 42 refs.

Steiner G: Diabetes and atherosclerosis. An overview. *Diabetes,* 30 (Suppl. 2):1–7, 1981.

A recent review of this poorly-understood diabetic complication with emphasis on recent data concerning diabetes, platelets and arterial smooth muscle cells. 109 refs.

Malone JI, VanCader TC and Edwards WC: Diabetic vascular changes in children. ***Diabetes,*** **26:673–679, 1977.**
154 diabetic children were evaluated by fluorescein angiography. The severity of the retinopathy increased with duration of diabetes; however, 13 percent of children had retinopathy after less than 1 year of diabetes. 15 refs.

Retinopathy

Rand LI: Recent advances in diabetic retinopathy. ***Am J Med,*** **70:595–602, 1981.**
In this brief but very informative review, the author describes recent advances in the treatment of diabetic retinopathy, including the indications for photocoagulation and vitrectomy. He also reviews the available data on vitreous fluorophometry and other newer techniques. 73 refs.

Liang JC and Goldberg MF: Treatment of diabetic retinopathy. ***Diabetes,*** **29:841–851, 1980.**
A brief, recent general review of the current management of diabetic retinopathy, written by ophthalmologists for internists. 106 refs.

Palmberg PF: Diabetic retinopathy. ***Diabetes,*** **26:703–709, 1977.**
A brief review of the social impact, staging, pathogenesis and treatment of diabetic retinopathy. 79 refs.

British Multicentre Photocoagulation Trial. Proliferative diabetic retinopathy: Treatment with xenon-arc photocoagulation. ***Br Med J,*** **1:739–741, 1977.**
100 patients with proliferative diabetic retinopathy underwent photocoagulation therapy of one eye, the other serving as a control. Visual acuity deteriorated less with photocoagulation in one subgroup of patients, and blindness was prevented to a significant degree. 10 refs.

British Multicentre Photocoagulation Trial. Photocoagulation in the treatment of diabetic maculopathy. ***Lancet,*** **2:1,110–1,113, 1975.**
76 patients with diabetic maculopathy received photocoagulation therapy to one eye only. Visual acuity was better in the treated eyes at one, two and three years. 8 treated eyes became blind compared to 18 controls. 14 refs.

Job D, Eschwege E, Guyot-Argenton C et al.: Effect of multiple

daily insulin injections on the course of diabetic retinopathy. ***Diabetes*****, 25:463–469, 1976.**
This study is a prospective, randomized trial of multiple versus single insulin injections in the control of diabetic retinopathy in 42 patients. The progression of retinopathy was less in the group receiving multiple injections; however, dropouts from the study make its statistical validity questionable. 47 refs.

Gerritzen FM: The course of diabetic retinopathy. ***Diabetes*****, 22:122–128, 1973.**
Serial retinal photographs were taken in 459 diabetics over 8 years. During this period, 48 percent of patients developed worse retinopathy, 38 percent remained unchanged and 44 percent improved. 11 refs.

Beaumont P and Hollows FC: Classification of diabetic retinopathy with therapeutic implications. ***Lancet*****, 1:419–425, 1972.**
Diabetic retinopathy is divided into four groups on the basis of fluorescein angiography, opthalmologic and biochemical evaluations. The authors conclude that the four entities have different prognostic implications. 51 refs.

Burditt AF, Caird FI and Draper GJ: The natural history of diabetic retinopathy. ***Q J Med*****, 37:303–317, 1968.**
This prospective study of diabetic retinopathy consisted of serial opthalmologic evaluations of over 2,000 patients in 1 clinic. The progression and incidence of retinopathy, including malignant retinopathy, were evaluated and related to age and duration of diabetes. 54 refs.

White NH, Waltman SR, Krupin T and Santiago JV: Reversal of abnormalities in ocular fluorophotometry in insulin-dependent diabetes after five to nine months of improved metabolic control. ***Diabetes*****, 31:80–85, 1982.**
Vitreous fluorophotometry, a method for measuring possible fluorescein leakage from retinal vessels, showed that abnormal fluorescein levels improved in 11 diabetics treated intensively but not in 25 treated conventionally. Among the 11 intensively treated patients, no improvement was noted in two with proliferative retinopathy. 32 refs.

Neuropathy

Clarke BF, Ewing DJ and Campbell IW: Diabetic autonomic neuropathy. ***Diabetologia*****, 17:195–212, 1979.**
An extensive, recent review of autonomic neuropathy, with emphasis on the clinical features and treatment of these disorders. 24 refs.

Hosking DJ, Bennett T and Hampton JR: Diabetic autonomic neuropathy. *Diabetes,* 27:1,043–1,054, 1978.
A concise review of these neglected disorders, with extensive literature review; no discussion of peripheral neuropathy. 133 refs.

Ellenberg M: Diabetic neuropathy: Clinical aspects. *Metabolism,* 25:1,627–1,655, 1976.
An exhaustive review of clinical aspects of both peripheral and autonomic diabetic neuropathy. 91 refs.

Goldstein F, Wirts CW and Kowlessor OD: Diabetic diarrhea and steatorrhea. *Ann Intern Med,* 72:215–218, 1970.
2 of 10 patients with diabetic diarrhea demonstrated small intestinal bacterial overgrowth and responded to specific antibiotic therapy. 18 refs.

Katz LA and Spiro HM: Gastrointestinal manifestations of diabetes. *N Engl J Med,* 275:1,350–1,361, 1966.
A review of gastrointestinal manifestations and complications of diabetes, with no new data. 88 refs.

Spritz N: Nerve disease in diabetes mellitus. *Med Clin North Am,* 62:787–798, 1978.
A brief, recent review of this topic. 51 refs.

Greyersen G: Diabetic neuropathy: Influence of age, sex, metabolic control and duration of diabetes on motor conduction velocity. *Neurology,* 17:972–980, 1967.
Motor conduction velocity was assessed in 145 randomly selected diabetics without other neuropathies. Motor conduction velocity decreased with duration of diabetes, especially in the younger patients; it was also lower in patients in poor metabolic control. 23 refs.

Colby AD: Neurologic disorders of diabetes mellitus. *Diabetes,* 14:424–429; 516–525, 1965.
A still current review of diabetic neuropathy, with emphasis on pathology, clinical manifestations and prognosis. 206 refs.

Sinha S, Munichoodappa CS and Kozak GP: Neuroarthropathy (Charcot joints) in diabetes mellitus. *Medicine,* 51:191–210, 1972.
An extensive review of Joslin Clinic patients with Charcot joints between 1949 and 1970. The authors describe the clinical characteristics of 101 such patients. 129 refs.

Fraser DM, Campbell IW, Ewing DI and Clarke BF: Mononeuropathy in diabetes mellitus. *Diabetes,* 28:96–101, 1979.

Diabetic mononeuropathy occurred in 51 patients; the most common sites of involvement were median (30 percent), ulnar (30 percent) and lateral popliteal nerves (16 percent), while cranial nerves accounted for 14 percent. Aside from median and ulnar neuropathies, the onset was acute. 35 refs.

Zorilla E and Kozak GP: Opthalmoplegia in diabetes mellitus. ***Ann Intern Med*, 67:968–976, 1967.**
33 episodes of opthalmoplegia were described in 24 diabetic patients. Third nerve palsy was unilateral in 15 and bilateral in 2; the remaining 7 patients had sixth nerve palsy. Pain occurred in 44 percent; diplopia was present in all. 27 refs.

Locke S, Lawrence DG and Legg MA: Diabetic amyotrophy. ***Am J Med*, 34:775–785, 1963.**
The clinical features of 20 patients with diabetic amyotrophy are described. 19 had pain, 18 complained of weakness; the symptoms were always bilateral. Muscle biopsy findings were fairly characteristic. 50 refs.

Nephropathy

Mauer SM, Steffes MW and Brown DM: The kidney in diabetes. ***Am J Med*, 70:603–612, 1981.**
The authors review the pathological aspects of clinical and experimental diabetic renal disease, with a brief comment on current approaches to the diabetic patient with renal failure. 97 refs.

Kussman MJ, Goldstein HH and Gleason RE: The clinical course of diabetic nephropathy. ***JAMA*, 236:1,861–1,863, 1976.**
Records of 112 insulin-dependent diabetics were analyzed. On average, diabetes was present 17 years before proteinuria developed; early renal failure appeared 2 years later, and severe renal failure 4 years later. 9 refs.

Mitchell JC: End-stage renal failure in juvenile diabetes mellitus. ***Mayo Clin Proc*, 52:281–288, 1977.**
5 year survival of 43 juvenile-onset diabetics receiving renal transplants was 58 percent. Neuropathy but few other sequelae improved after transplantation. 26 refs.

Shapiro FL, Kjellstrand CM and Goetz FC: End-stage diabetic nephropathy: A symposium. ***Kidney Int*, 6:Suppl. 1, 1–186, 1974.**
A thorough and exhaustive look at the problems of end-stage diabetic nephropathy, including vascular, metabolic and neurologic complications, dialysis, transplantation and the psy-

chosocial problems faced by diabetics with renal failure. Each article referenced separately.

Takazakura E, Nakamoto Y, Hayakawa H et al.: Onset and progression of diabetic glomerulosclerosis. A prospective study based on serial renal biopsies. ***Diabetes,*** **24:1–9, 1975.**
Of 162 diabetic patients undergoing renal biopsy, 23 had serial biopsies. The progression of lesions appeared to correlate with type of diabetes, control of blood glucose and age of onset rather than duration of diabetes. 27 refs.

Miscellaneous

DeLeiva A, Christlieb AR, Melby JC et al.: Big renin and biosynthetic defect of aldosterone in diabetes mellitus. ***N Engl J Med,*** **295:639–643, 1976.**
Two patients with diabetic hypoaldosteronism were studied; both proved to have a defect in renin synthesis, with increased plasma concentrations of "big renin," and a defect in aldosterone synthesis. 64 refs.

Hamby RI, Zoneraich S and Sherman L.: Diabetic cardiomyopathy. ***JAMA,*** **229:1,749–1,754, 1974.**
16 of 73 patients with idiopathic cardiomyopathy had diabetes. Autopsies on 3 of the diabetics revealed characteristic small vessel changes in the heart, found in only one of 28 nondiabetic patients with cardiomyopathy. 14 refs.

Waller BF, Palumbo PJ, Lie JT and Roberts WC: Status of the coronary arteries at necropsy in diabetes mellitus with onset after age 30 years. Analysis of 229 diabetic patients with and without clinical evidence of coronary heart disease and comparison to 183 control subjects. ***Am J Med,*** **69:498–506, 1980.**
This is a careful autopsy study of hearts from 229 diabetic patients (presumably Type II) with and without clinically apparent coronary artery disease, compared to those from 183 matched non-diabetic patients with coronary disease. Severe left-main narrowing was more common in the diabetics. 41 refs.

Muller SA and Winkelman RK: Necrobiosis lipoidica diabeticorum. ***Arch Dermatol,*** **93:272–281, 1966.**
171 patients with necrobiosis lipoidica diabeticorum were described. The frequency in diabetes was estimated at .3 percent. The histology of the lesions was different in diabetic and nondiabetic patients; 77 percent of the diabetic patients were female. Local steroids were occasionally helpful. 17 refs.

Oral Hypoglycemic Agents

Skillman TG and Feldman JM: The pharmacology of sulfonylureas. ***Am J Med*****, 70:361–372, 1981.**
The authors review the pharmacology of the common sulfonylureas, emphasizing the advantageous properties of "second-generation" drugs like glyburide, glipizide and glibornuride over the more familiar first generation drugs. 33 refs

Bressler R and Shen SW: Clinical pharmacology of oral antidiabetic agents. ***N Engl J Med*****, 296:493–497; 787–793; 1977.**
An excellent review of pharmacology of clinically used agents. The authors conclude that "At present oral hypoglycemic agents have no demonstrated useful role in the management of maturity-onset diabetes mellitus, asymptomatic or symptomatic." 48 refs.

Lebovitz HE and Feinglos MN: Sulfonylurea drugs: Mechanism of antidiabetic action and therapeutic usefulness. ***Diabetes Care*****, 1:189–198, 1978.**
A recent, readable review of sulfonylurea actions, which concludes that these drugs have a place, albeit small, in the therapy of noninsulin requiring diabetes. 95 refs.

Krall LP and Chabot VA: Oral hypoglycemic agent update. ***Med Clin North Am*****, 62:681–694, 1978.**
A current review of oral hypoglycemic agent pharmacology and the University Group Diabetes Program (UGDP)study, which concludes that they still have a place in therapy when used with caution. 68 refs.

Feinstein AR: An analytic appraisal of the UGDP study. ***Clin Pharmacol Ther*****, 12:167–191, 1971.**
A methodologic assessment of the UGDP study, which reveals several statistical flaws. The author does not draw any therapeutic conclusions from his analysis. 33 refs.

Karam JH, Martin SB and Forsham PH: Antidiabetic drugs after the UGDP. ***Curr Rev Pharmacol*****, 15:351–366, 1975.**
A review of the UGDP conclusions and the pharmacology of antidiabetic drugs. The authors recommend cautious evaluation of "second-generation" sulfonylurea drugs. 127 refs.

Singer DL and Hurwitz D: Long-term experience with sulfonylureas and placebo. ***N Engl J Med*****, 277:450–456, 1967.**
31 percent of 282 patients responded as well to placebo as to tolbutamide in this single-blind, long-term study; 17 percent of 302 patients responded as well to placebo as to chlorpropamide. 19 refs.

UGDP: Effects of hypoglycemic agents on vascular complications in patients with adult-onset diabetes. III. Clinical implications of UGDP results. *JAMA*, 218:1,400–1,410, 1971.
This evaluation of the UGDP mortality results suggested that ". . . Oral hypoglycemic agents should be employed with more caution than in the past." 18 refs.

University Group Diabetes Program: A study of the effects of hypoglycemic agents on vascular complications in patients with adult-onset diabetes. II. Mortality results. *Diabetes*, 19:suppl. 2, 787–830, 1970.
823 newly diagnosed diabetics were divided into 2 insulin treated groups, 1 tolbutamide treated group and 1 placebo group. Cardiovascular mortality was 12.7 in the tolbutamide group, versus 4.9 for placebo, and 6.2 and 5.9 in the two insulin groups. 34 refs.

Lev-Ran A: Trial of placebo in long-term chlorpropamide treated diabetics. *Diabetologia*, 10:197–200, 1974.
50 diabetic patients on chlorpropamide were put on placebo without their knowledge. In 27 patients, fasting blood glucose did not change; it decreased in 2 and increased in 20 patients. 15 refs.

Tomkins GM and Blood A: Assessment of the need for continued oral therapy in diabetics. *Br Med J*, 1:649–651, 1972.
A brief report demonstrating that blood glucose was not affected in 31 percent of 64 adult-onset diabetics when they were changed from a sulfonylurea or phenformin to placebo. 12 refs.

Hansen JM and Christensen LK: Drug interactions with oral sulfonylurea hypoglycemic drugs. *Drugs*, 13:24–34, 1977.
An important review of drugs which can interact with oral hypoglycemic agents, causing severe hypoglycemia. 72 refs.

Hypoglycemia (See Also Insulinoma)

Fajans SS and Floyd JC Jr.: Fasting hypoglycemia in adults. *N Engl J Med*, 294:766–772, 1976.
A nice review of recent concepts in etiology, classification and diagnosis. 8 refs.

Marks V: Hypoglycemia. II. Other causes. *Clin Endocrinol Metab*, 5:769–782, 1976.
A brief review of extrapancreatic tumor-related hypoglycemia, reactive and alcoholic hypoglycemia. 49 refs.

Hofeldt FD: Reactive hypoglycemia. ***Metabolism,*** **24:1,193–1,208, 1975.**
A complete review of this controversial topic, emphasizing its heterogeneity. 156 refs.

Arky RA and Arons DL: Hypoglycemia in diabetes mellitus. ***Med Clin North Am,*** **55:919–930, 1971.**
A short review of hypoglycemia occurring in the setting of diabetes. 68 refs.

Freinkel N and Metzger BE: Oral glucose tolerance curve and hypoglycemias in the fed state. ***N Engl J Med,*** **280:820–828, 1969.**
A review of the physiology and clinical features of hypoglycemia in the fed state. The authors discuss this entity in relation to post-gastrectomy and "functional" hypoglycemia, and early adult-onset diabetes. 98 refs.

Seltzer HS: Drug-induced hypoglycemia: A review based on 473 cases. ***Diabetes,*** **21:955–966, 1972.**
Case reports of 431 patients with drug-induced hypoglycemia are reviewed by the author, and data are included from 42 other patients. More than 80 percent of all episodes and all deaths were accounted for by alcohol in children or nondiabetics (174 cases) or sulfonylureas (220 cases). A further 71 cases were caused by salicylates, simultaneous use of two hypoglycemic agents or by potentiators of hypoglycemic drugs. 201 refs.

Service FJ and Palumbo PJ: Factitial hypoglycemia. ***Arch Intern Med,*** **134:336–340, 1974.**
The authors used an assay for insulin antibodies to differentiate three cases of factitious insulin administration from insulinoma. 26 refs.

Miller SI, Wallace RJ, Musher DM et al.: Hypoglycemia as a manifestation of sepsis. ***Am J Med,*** **68:649–654, 1980.**
Nine patients with severe hypoglycemia related to sepsis are described of whom six died. Six patients had a metabolic acidosis presumed due to excess lactate accumulation; the authors recommend close attention to this problem in septic patients. 54 refs.

MacCuish AC, Munro JF and Duncan LJP: Treatment of hypoglycemic coma with glucagon, intravenous dextrose and mannitol infusion in 100 diabetics. ***Lancet,*** **2:946–949, 1970.**
100 diabetic patients with hypoglycemia and neurologic dysfunction preventing oral intake received IV or IM glucagon,

then IV dextrose. 40 awakened after glucagon only; another 40 responded to dextrose; 19 remained unconscious despite elevated blood sugars. Most of the last patients awoke after IV mannitol infusions. 8 refs.

Rizza RA, Cryer PE and Gerich JE: Role of glucagon, catecholamines and growth hormone in human glucose counterregulation. Effects of somatostatin and combined α- and β-adrenergic blockade on plasma glucose recovery and glucose flux rates after insulin-induced hypoglycemia. *J Clin Invest*, 64:62–71, 1979.
The use of combined somatostatin, α- and β-blocker administration in 13 normal subjects allowed the authors to conclude that the enhanced gluconeogenesis in the Somogyi phenomenon after insulin-induced hypoglycemia is mediated primarily through increased glucagon secretion, rather than secretion of growth hormone or catecholamines. 57 refs.

DeFronzo RA, Andres R, Bledsoe TA et al.: A test of the hypothesis that the rate of fall in glucose concentration triggers counterregulatory hormonal responses in man. *Diabetes*, 26:445–452, 1977.
Increased growth hormone, catecholamine and cortisol blood levels occurred only after blood glucose reached 30 to 40 mg/dl below fasting levels in 5 normal subjects followed after sustained hyperglycemia. 34 refs.

Insulin Resistance

Olefsky JM and Kolterman OG: Mechanisms of insulin resistance in obesity and noninsulin-dependent (Type II) diabetes. *Am J Med*, 70:151–168, 1981.
A recent review of the mechanisms thought to be involved in the insulin resistance of obesity and Type II diabetes, with emphasis on abnormalities at the insulin receptor and post-receptor steps. 168 refs.

Kahn CR and Rosenthal AS: Immunologic reactions to insulin: Insullin allergy, insulin resistance and the autoimmune insulin syndrome. *Diabetes Care*, 2:283–295, 1979.
A recent, complete and readable review of these syndromes, with comments on the antigenicity of various insulin preparations, the measurement and effects of insulin antibodies and the syndrome of autoimmunity to insulin. 99 refs.

Davidson JK and DeBra DW: Immunologic insulin resistance. *Diabetes*, 27:307–318, 1978.

The authors treated 35 patients with immunologic resistance to regular beef insulin (mean dose: 550 units/day) with sulfated beef insulin. Treatment was successful in all but 1 patient; the mean insulin dose had decreased to 66 U/day by 3 months. 29 refs.

Mattsen JR, Patterson R and Roberts M: Insulin therapy in patients with systemic insulin allergy. ***Arch Intern Med,*** **135:818–821, 1975.**
Insulin sensitivity was demonstrated by skin testing in 15 patients with a history of insulin allergy; elevated IgE antibodies to insulin were found in 8 of 12 patients. Desensitization was effective in preventing allergic reactions in several patients. 19 refs.

Lieberman P, Patterson R, Metz R and Lucena G: Allergic reactions to insulin. ***JAMA,*** **215:1,106–1,112, 1971.**
Five patients who developed angioneurotic edema or urticaria after insulin use are described; all had previous local reactions and a history of discontinuing insulin, then resuming its use. Two patients were successfully desensitized. 13 refs.

Kahn CR, Flier JS, Bar RS et al.: The syndromes of insulin resistance and acanthosis nigricans. ***N Engl J Med,*** **294:739–745, 1976.**
Six patients with acanthosis nigricans and simultaneous hyperglycemia and hyperinsulinism are described. All had diabetic glucose tolerance tests and decreased insulin binding to receptors; this appears to be mediated by antireceptor antibodies in a subgroup of these patients. 35 refs.

Shipp JC, Cunningham RW, Russell RO et al.: Insulin resistance: Clinical features, natural course and effects of adrenal steroid treatment. ***Medicine,*** **44:165–186, 1965.**
The clinical features of 34 patients with insulin resistance (defined as requiring more than 200 units of insulin daily for more than 2 days) are described. Insulin resistance lasted less than a year in 75 percent of patients; 4 patients responded to steroid therapy with a decrease in insulin requirement. 79 refs.

Diabetic Ketoacidosis

Kreisberg RA: Diabetic ketoacidosis: New concepts and trends in pathogenesis and treatment. ***Ann Intern Med,*** **88:681–695, 1978.**
This article reviews newer information on ketoacidosis. 137 refs.

Alberti KGMM and Nattrass M: Severe diabetic ketoacidosis. ***Med Clin North Am*, 62:799–814, 1978.**
A concise review of recent studies. 101 refs.

Hockaday TDR and Alberti KGMM: Diabetic coma. ***Clin Endocrinol Metab.*** **1:751–788, 1972.**
A detailed clinical review of early studies. 143 refs.

Beigelman PM: Severe diabetic ketoacidosis—482 episodes in 257 patients; experience of 3 years. ***Diabetes*, 20:490–500, 1971.**
A classic article describing the clinical and biochemical characteristics of 340 episodes of diabetic ketoacidosis in 257 patients. A good review of earlier series is included. 54 refs.

Kitabchi AE, Ayyagari V, Guerra SMO et al.: The efficacy of low dose versus conventional therapy of insulin for treatment of diabetic ketoacidosis. ***Ann Intern Med*, 84:633–638, 1976.**
In the first prospective randomized study of low dose insulin in diabetic ketoacidosis, the authors studied 48 patients divided into low and high dose groups. Biochemical improvement was similar in the 2 groups, but 25 percent of the high dose patients developed hypoglycemia versus none of the low dose group. 22 refs.

Fisher JN, Shahshahani MN and Kitabchi AE: Diabetic ketoacidosis: Low-dose insulin therapy by various routes. ***N Engl J Med*, 297:238–241, 1977.**
IV, SQ and IM routes of low dose insulin administration were compared in 45 patients with diabetic ketoacidosis. All three routes were adequate, with initial IV therapy in all groups speeding the decrease in glucose and ketone bodies. 21 refs.

Alberti KGMM: Low-dose insulin in the treatment of diabetic ketoacidosis. ***Arch Intern Med*, 137:1,367–1,376, 1977.**
A review of recent literature supporting low-dose insulin infusions in ketoacidosis. 92 refs.

Padilla AJ and Loeb JN: "Low-dose" versus "high-dose" insulin regimens in the management of uncontrolled diabetes. A survey. ***Am J Med*, 63:843–848, 1977.**
A concise review of this argument, which concludes that there is not much difference between the two types of therapy. 52 refs.

Heber D, Molitch ME and Sperling MA: Low-dose continuous insulin therapy for diabetic ketoacidosis. ***Arch Intern Med*, 137:1,377–1,380, 1977.**
17 cases of diabetic ketoacidosis were randomized to low-dose

(infusion) or high-dose (subcutaneous injection) groups. No differences in glucose or hormonal responses were noted, but continuous low-dose insulin infusion was recommended because of convenience. 24 refs.

Barnes AJ, Bloom SR, Alberti KGMM et al.: Ketoacidosis in pancreatectomized man. ***N Engl J Med,*** **296:1,250–1,253, 1977.**
Insulin withdrawal in six juvenile-onset diabetics and four pancreatectomized patients produced hyperglycemia and hyperketonemia in both groups, not as marked in the pancreatectomized patients, suggesting that glucagon is not necessary for development of ketosis. 32 refs.

Beigelman PM: Potassium in severe diabetic ketoacidosis. ***Am J Med,*** **54:419–420, 1973.**
A brief editorial emphasizing the need for vigorous potassium replacement in the treatment of diabetic ketoacidosis. 12 refs.

Assal JP, Aoki TT, Manzano FM and Kozak GP: Metabolic effects of sodium bicarbonate in management of diabetic ketoacidosis. ***Diabetes,*** **23:405–411, 1974.**
Nine patients with diabetic ketoacidosis were given sodium bicarbonate plus insulin and saline. They displayed lower CSF pH after treatment than a previous group of patients treated with insulin and saline alone, and higher CSF osmolality, but the clinical course was no different. 14 refs.

Peterson L, Caldwell J and Hoffman J: Insulin adsorbance to polyvinylchloride surfaces with implications for constant infusion therapy. ***Diabetes,*** **25:72–74, 1976.**
An important in vitro study, demonstrating that albumin is not necessary in insulin infusion solutions if 50 ml of the infusate is washed through the tubing before beginning the infusion. 11 refs.

Gibby OM, Veale KEA, Hayes TM et al.: Oxygen availability from the blood and the effect of phosphate replacement on erythrocyte 2,3-diphosphoglycerate and haemoglobin-oxygen affinity in diabetic ketoacidosis. ***Diabetologia,*** **15:381–385, 1978.**
11 patients with diabetic ketoacidosis were treated with enough phosphorus to maintain normal plasma phosphate levels and restore 2,3-DPG levels to normal within 24 hours. This had no effect on indices of oxygen availability, compared to 10 patients treated without phosphorus; thus, they don't recommend phosphate in diabetic ketoacidosis. 19 refs.

Kanter Y, Gerson JR and Bessman AN: 2,3-diphosphoglycer-

ate, nucleotide phosphate and organic and inorganic phosphate levels during the early phases of diabetic ketoacidosis. ***Diabetes,*** **26:429–433, 1977.**
6 patients with diabetic ketoacidosis exhibited a marked decrease in serum inorganic phosphorus levels during treatment, while red cell 2,3-DPG levels remained low. The authors discuss the theoretical need for phosphate replacement in diabetic ketoacidosis. 22 refs.

Soler NG, Dixon K, Bennett MA et al.: Potassium balance during treatment of diabetic ketoacidosis. ***Lancet,*** **2:665–667, 1972.**
Potassium requirements were assessed during treatment of 25 patients with diabetic ketoacidosis. These ranged from 225 to 343 mEq per patient during the first 24 hours. 17 refs.

Guisado R and Arieff AI: Neurologic manifestations of diabetic comas: Correlation with biochemical alterations in the brain. ***Metabolism,*** **24:665–679, 1975.**
A detailed review of the reported neurologic manifestations of diabetic ketoacidosis and hyperosmolar nonketotic diabetic coma. The authors also speculate on the metabolic causes of coma and cerebral edema in these syndromes. 93 refs.

Clements RS Jr., Blumenthal SA, Morrison AD et al.: Increased cerebrospinal fluid pressure during treatment of diabetic ketosis. ***Lancet,*** **4:671–675, 1971.**
Cerebrospinal fluid pressure increased during therapy in five patients being treated for diabetic ketoacidosis, and was often associated with transient alterations in mental status. 19 refs.

Ohman JL Jr., Marliss EB, Aoki TT et al.: The cerebrospinal fluid in diabetic ketoacidosis. ***N Engl J Med,*** **284:283–290, 1971.**
Increased cerebrospinal fluid osmolality and normal or elevated pH were noted in six patients with diabetic ketoacidosis before treatment. These findings and the fall of CSF pH during treatment suggested that bicarbonate and rapid correction of osmolality both be used with great caution. 36 refs.

Nabarro JDN, Spencer AG and Stowers JM: Metabolic studies in severe diabetic ketosis. ***Q J Med,*** **21:225–248, 1952.**
A classic study of water and electrolyte requirements during recovery from diabetic ketoacidosis in 19 patients. 37 refs.

Hyperosmolar Coma

Podolsky S: Hyperosmolar nonketotic coma in the elderly diabetic. ***Med Clin North Am,*** **62:815–828, 1978.**

A brief, current review of recent literature on hyperosmolar coma, with emphasis on diagnosis and treatment in the elderly. 109 refs.

Gordon EE and Kabadi UM: The hyperglycemic hyperosmolar syndrome. ***Am J Med Sci,*** **271:253–268, 1976.**
A very good general review with no new data. 169 refs.

Foster DW: Insulin deficiency and hyperosmolar coma. ***Adv Intern Med,*** **19:159–173, 1974.**
A good brief review, with emphasis on pathophysiology, written before low-dose insulin became popular. 74 refs.

McCurdy DK: Hyperosmolar hyperglycemic nonketotic diabetic coma. ***Med Clin North Am,*** **54:683–699, 1970.**
A good early review of the syndrome, with particular attention paid to osmotic changes in body fluids. Data are included from 84 patients, of whom 34 died. 64 refs.

Arieff AI and Carroll HJ: Nonketotic hyperosmolar coma with hyperglycemia: Clinical features, pathophysiology, renal function, acid-base balance, plasma-cerebrospinal fluid equilibria and the effects of therapy in 37 cases. ***Medicine,*** **51:73–94, 1972.**
This report describes a careful metabolic evaluation of 34 patients experiencing 37 episodes of hyperosmolar coma before the era of low-dose insulin. 104 refs.

Gerich JR, Martin MM and Recant L: Clinical and metabolic characteristics of hyperosmolar nonketotic coma. ***Diabetes,*** **20:228–238, 1971.**
The authors compared 20 patients with the hyperosmolar nonketotic syndrome to 10 with ketoacidosis. The former group had lower plasma free fatty acid, growth hormone and cortisol levels, but higher serum osmolality and mortality. 48 refs.

Aireff AI and Carroll HJ: Cerebral edema and depression of sensorium in nonketotic hyperosmolar coma. ***Diabetes,*** **23:525–531, 1974.**
A correlation between depression of sensorium and plasma osmolality was found in 53 patients with hyperglycemia without ketosis. Cerebral edema did not occur if blood glucose was not acutely lowered below 250 mg/dl. 28 refs.

Maccario M: Neurological dysfunction associated with nonketotic hyperglycemia. ***Arch Neurol,*** **19:525–534, 1968.**
A good review of the types of neurologic dysfunction occurring in this syndrome, emphasizing that focal signs as well as stupor occur commonly. Data from seven patients are included. 73 refs.

Lactic Acidosis

Kreisberg RA: Lactate homeostasis and lactic acidosis. ***Ann Intern Med*****, 92:227–239, 1980.**
A complete, recent update of his earlier review on the subject, emphasizing the decline in importance of phenformin, and possible new therapies for this disorder. 96 refs.

Harken AH: Lactic acidosis. ***Surg Gynecol Obstet*****, 142:593–606, 1976.**
A good recent review, with emphasis on pathophysiology of excess lactate production. 146 refs.

Cohen RD: Disorders of lactic acid metabolism. ***Clin Endocrinol Metab*****, 5:613–625, 1976.**
A biochemically oriented review of lactate metabolism and lactic acidosis. 21 refs.

Oliva PB: Lactic acidosis. ***Am J Med*****, 48:209–225, 1970.**
The best and most comprehensive review of lactic acidosis currently available. 272 refs.

Luft D: Lactic acidosis in biguanide treated diabetics: A review of 330 cases. ***Diabetologia*****, 14:75–87, 1978.**
A comprehensive review of lactic acidosis in patients treated with phenformin, metformin and buformin. The overall mortality was 50 percent; poor prognostic indicators were advanced age, shock, high lactate levels and renal insufficiency. 175 refs.

Fulop M and Hoberman HD: Phenformin associated metabolic acidosis. ***Diabetes*****, 25:292–296, 1976.**
18 phenformin treated diabetic patients were studied, all of whom had elevated blood lactate levels. Many also had elevated 3-hydroxybutyrate levels, leading to the authors' recommendation that insulin and glucose should be used to treat many of these patients. 23 refs.

Alcoholic Ketosis

Fulop M and Hoberman HD: Alcoholic ketosis. ***Diabetes*****, 24:785–790, 1975.**
21 patients with severe alcoholic ketosis were studied, of whom 15 were not diabetic and 6 had mild postprandial hyperglycemia. Most patients benefitted from saline and glucose alone. 20 refs.

Cooperman MT, Davidoff F, Spark R and Pallotta J: Clinical studies of alcoholic ketoacidosis. ***Diabetes*****, 23:433–439, 1974.**

These authors describe seven episodes of alcoholic ketosis in six patients; all patients recovered quickly with glucose, saline and occasional bicarbonate. 35 refs.

Levy LJ, Duga J, Girgis M and Gordon EE: Ketoacidosis associated with alcoholism in nondiabetic subjects. ***Ann Intern Med,*** **78:213–219, 1973.**
Five alcoholic patients experiencing six episodes of nondiabetic ketoacidosis were studied. The ketosis was thought due to markedly enhanced adipose tissue lipolysis; therapy with glucose, fluid and bicarbonate was effective. 40 refs.

Miller PD, Heinig RE and Waterhouse C: Treatment of alcoholic acidosis. ***Arch Intern Med,*** **138:67–72, 1978.**
Glucose infusion decreased hydroxybutyrate faster than did saline in 10 patients being treated for 18 episodes of alcoholic ketosis, and resulted in marked hypophosphatemia; the authors recommend glucose and fluid alone for therapy. 39 refs.

Munro JF, Campbell IW, McCuish AC and Duncan LJP: Euglycemic diabetic ketoacidosis. ***Brit Med J,*** **2:578–580, 1973.**
17 patients in a series of 211 cases of "diabetic metabolic decompensation" had severe ketosis (bicarbonate less than 10 mEq/1) with blood sugars less than 300 mg/ml, for a total of 37 episodes. The patients were young, mostly female and had known insulin-dependent diabetes at the time of admission; alcohol was not implicated in the pathogenesis. 7 refs.

Islet Cell Tumors (See Also Zollinger-Ellison Syndrome, Gastrointestinal Diseases)

General

Holst JJ: Gut endocrine tumor syndromes. ***Clin Endocrinol Metab,*** **8:413–432, 1979.**
A brief review of the recent literature on the Vernon-Morrison, insulinoma and glucagonoma syndromes. 89 refs.

Walsh JH, Tompkins RK, Taylor IL et al.: Gastrointestinal hormones in clinical disease: Recent developments. ***Ann Intern Med,*** **90:817–828, 1979.**
A recent, readable review of gut hormone pathophysiology, with emphasis on the pancreatic cholera syndrome. The literature on glucagonomas and somatostatinomas is also reviewed. 98 refs.

Schein PS, DeLellis RA, Kahn CR et al. Islet cell tumors: Current concepts and management. *Ann Intern Med*, 79:239–257, 1973.
A wide-ranging review of islet cell tumors, with emphasis on insulinoma, gastrinoma and VIPoma. 169 refs.

Cubilla AL and Hajdu SI: Islet cell carcinoma of the pancreas. *Ann Pathol*, 99:204–207, 1975.
30 patients with pancreatic islet cell carcinomas were studied, of which 57 percent were men. The tumors were greater than 6 cm in diameter when discovered in 83 percent of cases. 87 percent were metastatic at the time of diagnosis; mean survival was 3.9 years; the 5 year survival was 65 percent. 25 refs.

Broder LE and Carter SK: Pancreatic islet cell carcinoma: I. Clinical features of 52 patients. *Ann Intern Med*, 79:101–107, 1973.
Of 52 patients with metastatic islet cell carcinoma, 79 percent had functioning tumors, most of them insulin-secreting. Median survival was about three years from onset of symptoms. 44 refs.

Broder LE and Carter SK: Pancreatic islet cell carcinoma. II. Results of therapy with streptozotocin in 52 patients. *Ann Intern Med*, 79:108–118, 1973.
The response of metastatic islet cell carcinoma to streptozotocin was assessed in 52 patients. Patients with insulinomas generally had some biochemical response to treatment, and mean survival for "responders" was more than twice as great as that of the "nonresponders." Toxicity included fatal renal failure in five patients. 43 refs.

Robins JM, Bookstein JJ, Oberman HA and Fajans SS: Selective angiography in localizing islet cell tumors of the pancreas. *Radiology*, 106:525–528, 1973.
26 patients with insulinomas were studied with selective pancreatic angiography; the overall detection rate was 38 percent. Only 3 of 16 tumors less than 1 cm in diameter were visualized. 10 refs.

Harrison TS, Child CG, Fry WJ et al.: Current surgical management of functioning islet cell tumors of the pancreas. *Ann Surg*, 178:485–493, 1973.
A good review of the surgical aspects of insulinoma management, with emphasis on the entity of "microscopic adenomatosis" with hyperinsulinism. Data from 35 patients are reviewed. 35 refs.

Larson LI: Mixed endocrine pancreatic tumors producing several peptide hormones. ***Am J Pathol,*** **79:271–279, 1975.**
7 of 24 endocrine pancreatic tumors were found to contain more than 1 hormone producing cell type, 11 contained 1 cell type, and 6 contained no recognizable endocrine cell type. The mixed tumors contained glucagon, insulin, gastrin and ACTH. 35 refs.

Insulinoma (See Also Hypoglycemia)

Fajans SS and Floyd JC: Diagnosis and medical management of insulinomas. ***Ann Rev Med,*** **30:313–329, 1979.**
A brief and readable review of this topic, with important information on the drugs that may be useful in treating hyperinsulinism. 31 refs.

Frerichs H and Creutzfeldt W: Hypoglycemia. I. Insulin-secreting tumors. ***Clin Endocrinol Metab,*** **5:747–767, 1976.**
A pathologically oriented review of insulinomas. 83 refs.

Service FJ, Dale AJD, Elveback LR et al.: Insulinoma: Clinical and diagnostic features of 60 consecutive cases. ***Mayo Clin Proc,*** **51:417–429, 1976.**
60 consecutive patients presenting with insulinoma from 1964 to 1975 were described. About 60 percent were women. All 51 patients who underwent prolonged fasting demonstrated symptomatic hypoglycemia relieved by glucose (Whipple's triad). About 80 percent of the tumors were single and benign; 10 percent multiple, often as part of MEN I and about 10 percent were malignant. 41 refs.

Shen SW: Disordered glucose and insulin metabolism in patients with insulinoma. ***Arch Intern Med,*** **135:668–672, 1975.**
Two patients with insulinomas responded abnormally to infusions of glucose and propranolol/epinephrine. The author recommends these studies in assessing abnormalities of β-cell responsiveness. 25 refs.

Edis AJ, McIlrath DC, VanHeerden JA et al.: Insulinoma—Current diagnosis and surgical management. ***Curr Probl Surg,*** **13(10):1–45, 1976.**
A detailed review of the surgical approach to the patient with insulinoma. 39 refs.

Shatney CH and Grage TB: Diagnostic and surgical aspects of insulinoma. ***Am J Surg,*** **127:174–185, 1974.**
A complete discussion of insulinoma surgery, including salient features of 27 patients. 47 refs.

Service FJ, Horwitz DL, Rubenstein AH et al.: C-peptide suppression test for insulinoma. ***J Lab Clin Med,*** **90:180–186, 1977.**
11 of 12 patients with insulinoma failed to suppress C-peptide levels during hypoglycemia induced by exogenous insulin infusions; the authors suggest this as a useful suppression test. 14 refs.

Turner RC and Harris E: Diagnosis of insulinomas by suppression tests. ***Lancet,*** **1:188–190, 1974.**
Fish insulin infusions were used to induce hypoglycemia in 12 patients with insulinoma, 4 of whom had normal fasting blood glucoses. Failure to suppress endogenous insulin was noted in all cases. 7 refs.

Alsever RN, Roberts JP, Gerber JG et al.: Insulinoma with low circulating insulin levels: The diagnostic value of proinsulin measurements. ***Ann Intern Med,*** **82:347–350, 1975.**
One patient with an insulinoma is described who had low levels of plasma insulin during hypoglycemia, but had simultaneously elevated proinsulin levels. These measurement may be of value in the occasional patient in whom inappropriate insulin levels are not present. 26 refs.

Turner RC, Lee ECG, Morris PJ et al.: Localization of insulinomas. ***Lancet,*** **1:515–518, 1978.**
Percutaneous catheterization of the veins draining the pancreas was used to localize small insulinomas in two patients; the authors recommend this procedure if arteriography does not localize the tumor. 19 refs.

Eastman RC, Come SE, Strewler GJ et al.: Adriamycin therapy for advanced insulinoma. ***J Clin Endocrinol Metab,*** **44:142–148, 1977.**
Remissions of several months were achieved using adriamycin in two patients with metastatic insulinomas refractory to streptozotocin. 17 refs.

Glucagonoma, Somatostatinoma and VIPoma

Friesen SR: Tumors of the endocrine pancreas. ***N Engl J Med,*** **306:580–590, 1982.**
A recent review of the APUD (amine-precursor uptake and decarboxylation) concept and its application to the clinical and pathologic syndromes of endocrine pancreas tumors. 108 refs.

Leichter SB: Clinical and metabolic aspects of glucagonoma. ***Medicine,*** **59:100–113, 1980.**

A complete, recent review of this syndrome, which summarizes clinical and biochemical features from 41 cases. 156 refs.

Kessinger A, Lemon HM and Foley JF: The glucagonoma syndrome and its management. *J Surg Oncol*, 9:419–424, 1977.
The authors review 12 documented and 22 probable cases of glucagonoma: clinical manifestations included diabetes, anemia, skin rash (necrolytic migratory erythema), stomatitis and other symptoms; these regress when the tumor is removed. 23 refs.

Mallinson CN, Bloom SR, Warin AP et al.: A glucagonoma syndrome. *Lancet*, 2:1–5, 1974.
Nine patients are described with the "glucagonoma syndrome," comprising necrolytic migratory erythema, stomatitis and diabetes. All had pancreatic tumors, four of which contained and secreted glucagon. 32 refs.

Swenson KH, Amon RB and Hanifin JM: The glucagonoma syndrome. A distinctive cutaneous marker of systemic disease. *Arch Dermatol*, 114:224–228, 1978.
The skin manifestations of necrolytic migratory erythema in one patient with the glucagonoma syndrome are described and compared to conditions with similar rashes. 18 refs.

Unger RH and Orci L: Glucagon and the A cell. Physiology and pathophysiology. *N Engl J Med*, 304:1518–1524; 1575–1580, 1981.
A recent review of A cell physiology and glucagon secretion, with comments on relevant aspects of diabetes, glucagonoma and isolated glucagon deficiency. 115 refs.

Ganda OP, Weir GC, Soeldner JS et al.: "Somatostatinoma": A somatostatin-containing tumor of the endocrine pancreas. *N Engl J Med*, 296:963–967, 1977 and 297:1,352–1,353, 1977.
A patient with hyperglycemia and a pancreatic tumor was found at operation to have a D cell tumor containing large amounts of somatostatin. Diabetes remitted after removal of the tumor. 40 refs.

Larsson LI, Hirsch MA, Holst JJ et al.: Pancreatic somatostatinoma: Clinical features and physiological implications. *Lancet*, 1:666–668, 1977.
The first reported case of a patient with somatostatinoma, presenting as diarrhea, steatorrhea, hypochlorhydria and glucose intolerance. 14 refs.

Axelrod L, Bush MA, Hirsch HJ and Loo SWH: Malignant

somatostatinoma: Clinical features and metabolic studies. ***J Clin Endocrinol Metab*, 52:886–896, 1981.**
A patient is described with a malignant somatostatinoma. She developed hyperglycemia, an IgG M-component reminiscent of multiple myeloma, and moderate ketosis; the tumor responded curiously to streptozotocin with an increase in plasma somatostatin levels. 39 refs.

Verner JV and Morrison AB: Endocrine pancreatic disease with diarrhea. ***Arch Intern Med,*** **133:492–500, 1974.**
The authors of the original description of this syndrome describe 1 case and review the clinical features of 54 additional cases. The predominant features were watery diarrhea, hypokalemia, hypochlorhydria, diabetes and hypercalcemia. 83 refs.

Jaffe BM, Kopen DF, DeSchryver-Kecskemeti K et al.: Indomethacin-responsive pancreatic cholera. ***N Engl J Med,*** **297:817–821, 1977.**
The possible mediation of the diarrhea in this syndrome by prostaglandin E is discussed and supported by the clinical response of one patient with a pancreatic tumor to indomethacin. 41 refs.

Diabetes in Pregnancy

Mintz DH, Skyler JS and Chez RA: Diabetes mellitus and pregnancy. ***Diabetes Care,*** **1:49–63, 1978.**
A concise general review of pregnancy in the diabetic, including discussions of perinatal mortality, fetal-maternal metabolism, dietary and insulin management and care of the infant. 114 refs.

Felig P: Body fuel metabolism and diabetes mellitus in pregnancy. ***Med Clin North Am*, 61:43–66, 1977.**
A complete review of this subject, emphasizing normal fuel metabolism during pregnancy, the effects of diabetes on pregnancy, and the management of pregnant diabetics. 129 refs.

Kitzmuller JL, Khartley JP, Younger MD et al: Diabetic pregnancy and perinatal morbidity. ***Am J Obstet Gynecol*, 131:560–580, 1978.**
A complete review of this subject, based on experience with 147 diabetic patients. Perinatal survival was 96.6%; the cesarean section rate was 55%; the incidences of respiratory distress syndrome, major congenital anomalies, and hypoglycemia were 7.6%, 9% and 47%, respectively. 103 refs.

Soller NG, Walsh CH and Malins JM: Congenital malformations in infants of diabetic mothers. ***Q J Med*, 45:303–313, 1976.**
Of 701 infants born to diabetic mothers, 8% had congenital malformations (three to four times the normal rate). These were fatal in 3.8%; most common were anencephaly, spina bifida, transposition of the great vessels, and sacral dysgenesis. 28 refs.

Gabby SG, Mestman JH, Freeman RK et al: Management and outcome of class A diabetes mellitus. ***Am J Obstet Gynecol*, 127:465–469, 1977.**
In 261 women with class A diabetes (normal fasting blood glucose and abnormal glucose tolerance tests during pregnancy), perinatal mortality was not higher than that of the general population when the patients were carefully monitored. 29 refs.

Tylson JE and Hock RA: Gestational and pregestational diabetes: An approach to therapy. ***Am J Obstet Gynecol*, 125:1,009–1,027, 1976.**
A recent, readable review of diabetes in pregnancy, with emphasis on the maintenance of euglycemia in all types of diabetes. 130 refs.

Adashi EY, Pinto H and Tyson JE: Impact of maternal euglycemia on fetal outcome in diabetic pregnancy. ***Am J Obstet Gynecol*, 133:268–274, 1979.**
Careful control of blood glucose was attempted in 81 diet-controlled and 32 insulin-dependent diabetic pregnant women. Infant mortality was zero; macrosomia, neonatal hypoglycemia and congenital malformations were common in the diet-controlled group. 19 refs.

Freinkel N: Of pregnancy and progeny. ***Diabetes*, 29:1,023–1,035, 1980.**
An interesting, recent review of maternal-fetal metabolic relationships during pregnancy in the diabetic. 154 refs.

Jovanovic L, Druzin M and Peterson CM: Effect of euglycemia on the outcome of pregnancy in insulin-dependent diabetic women as compared with normal control subjects. ***Am J Med*, 71:921–927, 1981.**
Near-normal glycemic control was achieved in 52 diabetic women using intensive insulin therapy plus home blood glucose monitoring during pregnancy. Babies from diabetic mothers experienced no respiratory distress or congenital anomalies, and there was no fetal loss. 43 refs.

Rudolf MCJ, Coustan DR, Sherwin RS et al: Efficacy of the insulin pump in the home treatment of pregnant diabetics. *Diabetes*, 30:891–895, 1981.
Seven pregnant diabetics were treated with continuous subcutaneous insulin infusions at home for the last part of their pregnancies in this uncontrolled study. Near normal glucose indices and glycosylated hemoglobin levels were obtained, and the infants were all healthy. Pregnancy in diabetics may eventually become the first indication for prolonged insulin infusion therapy. 14 refs

Obesity

General

Mann GV: The influence of obesity on health. *N Engl J Med,* 291:178–185; 226–232; 1974.
The author reviews the possible causes of obesity, its assessment, and side effects, including hypertension and coronary disease. He pessimistically reviews the available treatment options as well. 138 refs.

Bray GA and Gallagher TF Jr.: Manifestations of hypothalamic obesity in man: A comprehensive investigation of eight patients and a review of the literature. *Medicine,* 54:301–330, 1975.
The authors describe eight patients with various hypothalamic lesions in whom secondary obesity developed. Tumors were the most common cause, followed by trauma and inflammatory disease. They review the literature thoroughly. 355 refs.

Mayer J: Some aspects of the problem of regulation of food intake and obesity. *N Engl J Med,* 274:610–616; 662–673; 722–731; 1966.
A masterful review by a leading nutritionist. It covers the diagnosis of obesity, hunger regulation, genetic factors and treatment of obesity. 139 refs.

Medical Therapy

Bistrian BR: Recent developments in the treatment of obesity with particular reference to semistarvation ketogenic regimens. *Diabetes Care,* 1:379–384, 1978.
A brief review of semistarvation diets in the treatment of obesity, including the author's own "protein-sparing modified fast." 31 refs.

Genuth SM, Castro JH and Vertes V: Weight reduction in obesity by outpatient semistarvation. ***JAMA*****, 230:987–991, 1974.**
A semistarvation weight reduction program was used in 75 patients with massive obesity. 60 percent lost more than 40 lbs; the mean loss was 85 lbs; no serious side effects were noted. Follow-up weight changes were not noted. 22 refs.

Stunkard A: New therapies for the eating disorders. Behavior modification of obesity and anorexia nervosa. ***Arch Gen Psychiatry*****, 26:391–398, 1972.**
The author reviews the use of behavior modification psychotherapy in the treatment of both moderate and severe obesity; he argues that this therapy has been shown to be an improvement over other types of treatment. 38 refs.

Sims EAH, Horton ES and Salans LB: Inducible metabolic abnormalities during development of obesity. ***Annu Rev Med*****, 22:235–250, 1971.**
The authors review their work on experimental human obesity, in which they found that fat cell size (but not number) increased, as did plasma triglyceride, cholesterol and plasma insulin; glucose tolerance descreased in some but not all weight gainers. 62 refs.

Surgical Therapy

VanItallie TB, Bray GA, Faloon WW et al.: Symposium on surgical treatment of morbid obesity. ***Am J Clin Nutr*****, 33:356–530, 1980.**
An entire issue of this journal is devoted to a report of an NIH consensus conference held in December, 1978. This is the most complete contemporary review available of most aspects of surgical treatment of morbid obesity. Many refs.

The Danish Obesity Project: Randomised trial of jejunoileal bypass versus medical treatment in morbid obesity. ***Lancet*****, 2:1,255–1,258, 1979.**
Morbidly obese subjects were divided into groups with medical (66) or surgical (130) treatment. The patients treated surgically lost a median of 43 kg in 2 years, compared to 6 kg in the medically treated group. No deaths were noted in the surgical group; however, 6 percent had wound dehiscence, and 2 patients had severe hepatic dysfunction. 36 refs.

Halverson JD, Wisel L, Wazna MF and Ballinger WF: Jejunoileal bypass for morbid obesity. A critical appraisal. ***Am J Med*****, 64:461–475, 1978.**

Of 100 patients who received this operation, 5 died during the follow-up period: 3 from liver failure, 1 from pulmonary embolus and 1 with severe cachexia. 19 percent required restoration of intestinal continuity, and 58 percent had what the authors call major complications. 66 refs.

Faloon WW, ed: Symposium on jejunoileostomy for obesity. ***Am J Clin Nutr*, 30:1–129, 1977.**
A complete issue is devoted to papers on this operation and its use in obesity, including its success rates, metabolic effects, hepatic effects, nephrolithiasis, enteropathy, operative considerations and psychologic considerations. Many refs.

Bray GA, Barry RE, Benfield JR et al.: Intestinal bypass operation as a treatment for obesity. ***Ann Intern Med*, 85:97–109, 1976.**
This report of a UCLA conference reviews the results of ileojejunal bypass surgery, its psychiatric effects, and the surgical and medical complications of the procedure. 61 refs.

Parfitt AM, Miller MJ, Frame B et al.: Metabolic bone disease after intestinal bypass for treatment of obesity. ***Ann Intern Med*, 89:193–199, 1978.**
52 patients were assessed after intestinal bypass. Accelerated loss of bone was noted, and was associated with low plasma 25-hydroxycholecalciferol, suggesting that the patients malabsorbed vitamin D and calcium. 36 refs.

MISCELLANEOUS ENDOCRINE DISORDERS

Ectopic Hormone Production (General)

Imura H: Ectopic hormone syndromes. ***Clin Endocrinol Metab*, 9:235–260, 1980.**
A recent review in which the author discusses general aspects of ectopic hormone production, followed by brief descriptions of several common syndromes. 77 refs.

Blackman MR, Rosen SW and Weintraub BD: Ectopic hormones. ***Adv Intern Med*, 23:85–113, 1978.**
A recent review of this topic with much new information on ectopic production of pituitary peptides and glycoproteins. 101 refs.

Smith LH: Ectopic hormone production. ***Surg Gynecol Obstet*, 141:443–453, 1975.**
A brief but well-referenced review of the various ectopic hormone syndromes. 203 refs.

Rees LH and Ratcliffe JC: Ectopic hormone production by nonendocrine tumours. ***Clin Endocrinol,*** **3:263–299, 1974.**
A detailed review of most of the known ectopic hormone syndromes. 181 refs.

Liddle GW, Nicholson WE, Island DP et al.: Clinical and laboratory studies of ectopic humoral syndromes. ***Recent Prog Horm Res,*** **25:283–314, 1969.**
An extensive review of ectopic hormone-producing tumors. 97 refs.

Multiple Endocrine Neoplasia (MEN) Syndromes

General

Tischler AS, Dichter MA, Biales B and Greene LA: Neuroendocrine neoplasms and their cells of origin. ***N Engl J Med,*** **296:919–925, 1977.**
A concise review of the APUD cell hypothesis of Pearse. 25 refs.

Weichert RF III:The neural ectodermal origin of the peptide-secreting endocrine glands. ***Am J Med,*** **49:232–241, 1970.**
The author briefly reviews this concept in relation to the MEN syndromes and ectopic hormone production by tumors. 194 refs.

Harrison TS and Thompson NW: Multiple endocrine adenomatosis—I and II. ***Curr Probl Surg,*** **12:1–51, 1975 (August).**
An extensive review of the multiple endocrine neoplasia syndromes, with an emphasis on surgical management. 187 refs.

Schimke RN: Multiple endocrine adenomatosis syndromes. ***Adv Intern Med,*** **21:249–265, 1976.**
A brief review of the various manifestations of patients with MEN 1 and MEN 2. 64 refs.

MEN 1

Yamaguchi K, Kameya T and Abe K: Multiple endocrine neoplasia type 1. ***Clin Endocrinol Metab,*** **9:261–284, 1980.**
A recent review of this complicated syndrome, with emphasis on clinical features and management. 71 refs.

Ballard HS, Frame B and Hartsock RJ: Familial multiple endocrine adenoma-peptic ulcer complex. ***Medicine,*** **43:481–516, 1964.**

The clinical features of a 42 member family with the MEN type 1 syndrome and 72 additional cases of MEN 1 are reviewed. A thorough review of the older literature. 148 refs.

Lamers CB, Buis JT and VanTongeren J: Secretion-stimulated serum gastrin levels in hyperparathyroid patients from families with multiple endocrine adenomatosis type 1. *Ann Intern Med,* 86:719–724, 1977.
Of 23 patients with hyperparathyroidism in MEN 1 families, 9 had extreme increases in gastrin in response to secretin. All nine had Zollinger-Ellison syndrome. 19 refs.

Veldhuis JD, Green JE III, Kovacs E et al.: Prolactin-secreting pituitary adenomas. Association with multiple endocrine neoplasia, type I. *Am J Med,* 67:830–837, 1979.
The authors describe two patients in whom prolactinomas were the initial presentation of MEN 1, leading in turn to the evaluation of a very large kindred with the syndrome. The pituitary histology was similar to that of sporadic prolactinomas. 53 refs.

Farid NR, Buehler S, Russell NA et al.: Prolactinomas in familial multiple endocrine neoplasia syndrome type I. Relationship to HLA and carcinoid tumors. *Am J Med,* 69:874–880, 1980.
The authors describe four families with MEN I associated with prolactinomas. They suggest that prolactinomas are an integral part of the syndrome, and that thymic carcinoids may be an additional tumor associated with the syndrome. 50 refs.

MEN 2

Sizemore GW, Heath H III and Carney JA: Multiple endocrine neoplasia type 2. *Clin Endocrinol Metab,* 9:299–315, 1980.
The authors discuss the tumors which comprise the MEN 2a syndrome, after a brief discussion of MEN 2b. 59 refs.

Steiner AL, Goodman AD and Powers SR: Study of a kindred with pheochromocytoma, medullary thyroid carcinoma, hyperparathyroidism and Cushing's Disease: Multiple endocrine neoplasia type 2. *Medicine,* 47:371–409, 1968.
A family of 186 members with a high incidence of MEN 2 is described. The authors also review the relevant literature. 147 refs.

Keiser HR, Beaven MA, Doppman J et al.: Sipple's syndrome: Medullary thyroid carcinoma, pheochromocytoma and para-

thyroid disease: Studies in a large family. ***Ann Intern Med,*** **78:561–579, 1973.**
An NIH conference on MEN 2, in which the clinical, biochemical and radiographic features and the surgical management of patients with this syndrome are reviewed. 59 refs.

Lips CJ, Minder WH, Leo JR et al.: Evidence of multicentric origin of the multiple endocrine neoplasia syndrome type 2 (Sipple's syndrome) in a large family in the Netherlands. Diagnostic and therapeutic implications. ***Am J Med,*** **64:569–578, 1978.**
Six patients with MEN 2a are described, many of whom had multiple and bilateral pheochromocytomas and medullary thyroid carcinomas. The authors feel that these findings dictate a more radical surgical approach. 30 refs.

Carney JA, Sizemore GW and Tyce GM: Bilateral adrenal medullary hyperplasia in multiple endocrine neoplasia, Type 2. The precursor of bilateral pheochromocytoma. ***Mayo Clin Proc,*** **50:3–10, 1975.**
A patient with MEN 2 underwent bilateral adrenalectomy when high urinary levels of VMA were noted. The adrenal histology showed diffuse, non-nodular medullary hyperplasia. The authors suggest that this may be a precursor of pheochromocytoma in MEN 2. 34 refs.

Khairi MRA, Dexter RN, Burzynski NJ and Johnston CC: Mucosal neuroma, pheochromocytoma and medullary thyroid carcinoma: Multiple endocrine neoplasia type 3. ***Medicine,*** **54:89–112, 1975.**
The authors describe four patients with this syndrome, sometimes labeled type 2b in the literature. They also review the clinical features of 37 other patients from the literature. 81 refs.

Carney JA and Hayles AB: Alimentary tract manifestations of multiple endocrine neoplasia type 2b. ***Mayo Clin Proc,*** **52:543–548, 1977.**
The gastrointestinal manifestations of MEN 2b (elsewhere known as type 3) appear to be due to diffuse ganglioneuromatosis of the gastrointestinal tract. The gastrointestinal symptoms of 17 patients with this syndrome are discussed in relation to the relevant pathology. 15 refs.

The Carcinoid Syndrome

Teitelbaum SL: The carcinoid. A collective review. ***Am J Surg,*** **123:564–572, 1972.**

A short and readable review of carcinoid tumors and the carcinoid syndrome, with emphasis on surgical rather than endocrinologic aspects. 82 refs.

Grahame-Smith DG: The carcinoid syndrome. ***Am J Cardiol,*** **21:376–387, 1968.**
A brief review of the syndrome by the author of a recent textbook on the subject. He reviews the biochemistry, clinical features, diagnosis and treatment of the syndrome. 77 refs.

Davis Z, Moertel CG and McIlrath DC: The malignant carcinoid syndrome. ***Surg Gynecol Obstet,*** **137:637–644, 1973.**
Of 94 patients with malignant tumors and elevated urinary 5-hydroxyindoleacetic acid excretion, 2 had medullary thyroid cancer, 1 had lung oat-cell cancer and 91 had malignant carcinoids. Of these, 87 percent arose in the small intestine. Cutaneous flushing occurred in 65 percent; diarrhea in 75 percent and cardiac involvement in 20 percent. The median survival after the first flush was 38 months. 9 refs.

Sanders RJ and Axtell HK: Carcinoids of the gastrointestinal tract. ***Surg Gynecol Obstet,*** **199:369–380, 1964.**
A concise review of the older literature on intestinal carcinoid tumors and the carcinoid syndrome. 227 refs.

MacDonald RA: Study of 356 carcinoids of the gastrointestinal tract: Report of four new cases of the carcinoid syndrome. ***Am J Med,*** **21:867–878, 1956.**
Pathologic findings are reviewed from a large series of gastrointestinal carcinoid tumors. Of these, 58 percent were in the appendix. Of 146 extra-appendiceal tumors, 67 percent showed some degree of invasiveness. A high incidence of gastric and duodenal ulcers was noted. 64 refs.

Godwin JD II: Carcinoid tumors. An analysis of 2,837 cases. ***Cancer,*** **36:560–569, 1975.**
In these cases, reviewed retrospectively, about 44 percent of the tumors were appendiceal, 15 percent rectal, 11 percent ileal and 10 percent pulmonary. Lowest survival rates were for tumors of the stomach and intestine, while appendiceal tumors were probably never fatal. 30 refs.

Plonk JW and Feldman JM: Carcinoid arthropathy. ***Arch Intern Med,*** **134:651–654, 1974.**
Three of five patients with carcinoid syndrome complained of arthralgias, and four of five had characteristic skeletal changes, consisting of loss of bone density near the phalangeal

joints, cystic areas in the phalanges and erosion of the interphalangeal joint articular surfaces. 11 refs.

Roberts WC and Sjoerdsma A: The cardiac disease associated with the carcinoid syndrome (carcinoid heart disease). ***Am J Med,*** **36:5–34, 1964.**
An older and classic study of carcinoid heart disease in 17 patients with metastatic carcinoid tumors. Nine patients had heart disease. Most patients had a harsh, loud, systolic murmur at the upper left sternal border; pathologically, tricuspid regurgitation and pulmonic stenosis were the most common lesions. 47 refs.

Legha SS, Valdivieso M, Nelson RS et al: Chemotherapy for metastatic carcinoid tumors: Experiences with 32 patients and a review of the literature. ***Cancer Treat Rep,*** **61:1,699–1,703, 1977.**
A retrospective review of the results of treatment was performed for 32 patients with metastatic carcinoid tumors. The results were unimpressive, with adriamycin showing the most partial responses (five of seven patients). 13 refs.

Mengel CE: Therapy of the malignant carcinoid syndrome. ***Ann Intern Med,*** **62:587–602, 1965.**
An older but still useful review of surgical, medical and dietetic therapy in the palliative treatment of patients with the malignant carcinoid syndrome. 98 refs.